"Uncertainty, morning sickness, and anxiety suddenly turn to hope and direction in *A Catholic Mother's Companion to Pregnancy*, a book that will comfort, guide, and inspire you during your pregnancy."

Donna-Marie Cooper O'Boyle
Host of EWTN's *Everyday Blessings for Catholic Moms*

"Sarah Reinhard combines insight and humor to create yet another must-have book for Catholic moms. Whether this is your first pregnancy or your tenth, you'll find *A Catholic Mother's Guide to Pregnancy* to be an invaluable resource."

Jennifer Fulwiler
Blogger at *ConversionDiary.com*

"Sarah Reinhard takes the reader by the hand and walks her through the amazing process that is pregnancy. Never hesitating to explore both the challenges and the joys of this season of life, Sarah has created the guide to pregnancy that Catholic women have been waiting for."

Hallie Lord
Author of *Style, Sex, and Substance*

"Speaks to the hopes, fears, and love that come with nurturing a new life. This treasure of a book truly is a companion for expectant moms and its words of wisdom and encouragement will help readers mature in faith just as their baby matures in the womb."

Kate Wicker
Author of *Weightless: Making Peace with Your Body*

"To bring a new life into the world is the ultimate journey, so why not make it a spiritual journey? In *A Catholic Mother's Companion to Pregnancy*, Sarah Reinhard invites us to experience pregnancy and birth through the prism of our Catholic faith. Week by week, we marvel at what God has created within us, cling to him every step of the way for strength and consolation, and yearn for the moment when we will bring our long-awaited bundle of joy to the baptismal font to join the family of God. This book is a great journey companion for every Catholic mom-to-be. I sure wish I had it when I was pregnant with my four boys!"

Elizabeth Ficocelli
Author of *Seven from Heaven*

A Catholic Mother's Companion to Pregnancy

Walking with Mary *from* Conception to Baptism

SARAH A. REINHARD

Foreword by Lisa M. Hendey

ave maria press AmP notre dame, indiana

Founded in 1865, Ave Maria Press is a ministry of the United States Province of Holy Cross.

www.avemariapress.com

Paperback: ISBN-10 1-59471-298-0 ISBN-13 978-1-59471-298-2

E-book: ISBN-10 1-59471-351-0 ISBN-13 978-59471-351-4

Cover image "Holy Mother Mary" © 2011 Cecille Creations, www.cecillecreations.com

Cover and text design by John R. Carson.

Printed and bound in the United States of America.

Library of Congress Cataloging-in-Publication Data is available.

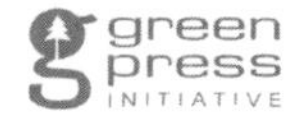

To Ali and Susie

Contents

Foreword

IT WAS COMPLETELY ON A WHIM THAT I REGISTERED CatholicMom.com in 2000. As the mother of two young sons, married to Greg, the love of my life (then a non-Catholic), I recall feeling completely overwhelmed not only by my motherly and spousal duties, but especially by the responsibility of raising our children in the Catholic faith.

So my motivations for buying a "dummies" computer book and starting a small website were largely selfish: I was desperate for support, encouragement, and information relevant to my vocation as a mother, especially a Catholic mother. This uniquely human desire to relate and to be in communion with one another never ceases to amaze me. Today I count most of the women with whom I connected back in those early days as dear friends. Many of them have gone on to become contributors to CatholicMom.com—a resource that welcomes hundreds of thousands of women from close to two hundred countries around the globe into a daily dialogue about the things that matter most in our lives. Together we have watched our babies be born and our children grow, we have prayed with and for one another, and we have done our very best to mentor the new moms who have come into our ever-blossoming fold.

These many years later, I still wake up each day and head anxiously to my desk with a joy for this mission that has become my life's work. While the ways in which our Church reaches out to us have developed and diversified over the centuries, her message remains as timeless as always. Although Catholic parents may have new trials and possibilities to face that are born of an ever-advancing technological culture, many of the fears, questions, delights, and joys we hold in our hearts are the same ones faced by our parents and grandparents.

As wives and single women, as stay-at-home moms and nine-to-fivers, as mothers and grandmothers, and especially as Catholics and women of faith, we are on a mission: to know, love, and serve God, to share his loving care with our family and friends, and to enjoy life with him forever in heaven. These are lofty goals that require a daily recommitment! This mission demands of us our very best. And to be at our best, we need all the help, support and encouragement we can find.

That is why I am thrilled to join force with my friends and colleagues at Ave Maria Press to create the CatholicMom.com book series to support you in your life's mission. We aim to educate, uplift, and inspire you with resources that are engaging and authentically Catholic. It's our great hope that these books, complemented by what we offer at CatholicMom.com, will nurture your heart, mind, body, and soul by addressing the cares that make motherhood more than a mere status and recognize it as the vocation that it is.

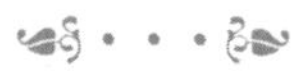

While it's hard for me to recall the exact moment I learned that I was pregnant for the first time, I can vividly recall the mix of emotions I felt as I glanced down at a positive pregnancy test. Shock and fear brought tears to my eyes that were only later soothed by the great joy my husband felt at our news. Unbeknownst to me, he had purchased a pregnancy test a few weeks prior "just in case." While I focused on my busy career, he daydreamed about his first child.

It took a few weeks for me to come into the joyful place Greg inhabited almost instantly. How I wish now—these twenty-some years later—that a book like the one you're holding had been available then. Sarah is a dear friend, and I rejoice that her companion for pregnancy, childbirth, and baptism is the inaugural title in the CatholicMom.com series. How fitting that a spiritual resource for pregnancy, childbirth, and baptism should give birth to a new line of resources for women anticipating, engaged in, or pondering the joys of motherhood.

What a companion you will find in Sarah! For me, she has been a friend, a role model, and a prayer warrior, and her work on behalf of the moms we serve at CatholicMom.com has been enthusiastic, innovative, and tireless. Sarah is the girlfriend who holds your hand throughout your pregnancy, labor and delivery, and through the celebration of your precious baby's baptism. But even more wonderful is the relationship Sarah invites you into with a loving Trinity, our Blessed Mother, and the communion of saints who have walked this earthly path and who intercede on our behalf as we travel through this temporal life.

Since I know and love Sarah, when I read this book I hear her wonderful voice in my head, offering practical counsel and making real and tangible those spiritual joys that fill our hearts. By the time you have enjoyed and prayed your way through *A Catholic Mother's Companion to Pregnancy*, your life will have been changed and blessed in ways you can only begin to imagine. Please know that you, your baby, and your family are in our prayers each step of the way!

Lisa M. Hendey

Preface

I NEVER THOUGHT I'D BE A MOTHER. IT WASN'T PART of the grand plan for my life, and even when I was baptized and confirmed a Catholic, I didn't see motherhood as something I wanted to do. I found it impossible to imagine myself as a mom. I had never wanted children of my own, and though my future nieces and nephews were cute, they weren't really relatable.

When I got married, I hoped for my husband's sake that we would have children. I knew that he loved kids, and I saw how kids loved him back.

All the same, I wasn't sure about the whole motherhood thing.

My first Mother's Day as a wife was also my first as a mom—I took a pregnancy test that afternoon. Now, eight years and three kids later, I can barely remember what I used to do in the evenings.

As I write this, I'm fresh off my third pregnancy, labor and birth, and Baptism. My son interrupts my writing to nurse, and my two older children interrupt with requests for juice, snacks, and attention.

This book is for you if you're pregnant with your first . . . or your fifth. I hope this companion helps you appreciate your time during pregnancy and through your baby's Baptism for the opportunity it is. Not only are you growing a human being and bringing him or her into the world, but you are also becoming a new person. Whether this is your first pregnancy or your fifth, this is the first time you've been down this path this way as the person you are right now.

Use this book as you would your favorite devotional. Write in the margins. Jot notes and dog-ear the pages. Make it your own.

Part one is a weekly journey through your pregnancy. After a brief reflection on what's happening with you and/or your baby, we'll reflect on a mystery of the Rosary. We will then discuss a small step you can take to integrate your Catholic faith into this experience and highlight a faith focus. Each chapter ends with a prayer that I encourage you to pray and even personalize so that you grow deeper in faith as your baby grows inside of you.

Part two examines labor and birth. In addition to a brief overview and some tips on preparing for each of these events, I offer some advice on incorporating spirituality into this special and challenging time. You'll learn how labor and birth lend themselves to prayer, and how they can help each of us grow in our understanding of the paschal mystery.

In part three, you'll find resources for Baptism, including an overview, preparation, and reflections. You'll want to explore this section before your baby's born and tap into the resources so that you're ready for this important day.

This is a very special and, in many ways, sacred time for you. Please know that, though we may never meet or talk, I am praying for you and your baby.

PART ONE

Weekly Journey through Pregnancy

PREGNANCY DOESN'T HAPPEN ALL AT ONCE, BUT eases itself into our being. We might be torn apart by sickness and stretch marks, but this prepares us for the many more grueling hours of motherhood ahead of us.

Pregnancy happens week by week, so we'll be journeying together toward that baby, the one we're praying you'll hold in your arms. As with any adventure, things don't always turn out the way you expect or plan.

This section includes a weekly approach to your pregnancy. The introduction to each chapter considers what's probably happening to your bodies—yours and baby's. It's not meant to replace any of the usual books and is only a very brief and incomplete approach. Because your baby's a person, right from the beginning, I'll be using gender pronouns, such as "he" or "she," instead of "it."

In the "Walking with Mary" sections, you'll find a mystery of the Rosary, and we'll reflect on it in light of where you are in your pregnancy. In the forty weeks of pregnancy, we can reflect on almost every mystery twice! "One Small Step" is meant to encourage you with a faith-related task you can complete each week. The "Faith Focus" in each week's chapter will highlight and explain an element of our Catholic faith. Since it is my prayer that you'll grow in your love for God as your baby grows inside of you, each chapter will close with a prayer to foster your conversation with God.

Throughout this section, you'll also find some features that focus on some of the difficult topics of pregnancy. In some ways, they don't "fit" the glowing and lovely idea of pregnancy, but they *are* very real. I asked some talented women to contribute, because some of these topics are beyond my range of experience. I wanted you to have a place to turn that was Catholic. If you find yourself in one of these situations during your pregnancy, I wanted to be able to offer you support—so often, these topics are taboo, silent, undiscussed. If you choose not to read them, I won't blame you, but they are there if you need them.

Don't wait until later in your pregnancy to read part two: "Labor and Birth," and part three: "Baptism." There are tips and tools included in those sections that will serve you well as you prepare for the end of your pregnancy.

Before we embark together on the adventure of pregnancy, let's offer a prayer that we can accept God's will and hold tight to Mother Mary's hand through the highs and lows of this grand adventure.

• • •

Mother Mary, walk with me through my pregnancy. Help me turn to your son with my fears and anxieties, annoyances and hardships. Guide me in the path to accepting God's will for my life and for this pregnancy. Pray for me, Mary, and hold me throughout the trials and joys ahead. Amen.

CHAPTER 1

The First Five Weeks (Fetal Age: 1–3 Weeks)

IT'S SO EARLY IN YOUR PREGNANCY THAT YOU MIGHT not feel any differently. By this point, you haven't even missed a period. Then again, that ongoing longing for your pillow and the queasy nausea that's been haunting you might suddenly make sense.

While you're going about your usual business with the idea of a baby feeling more like a theory than a reality, your baby has already embedded himself in your uterus. Though he may just seem to be a "blob," everything he needs to be a complete human being is in place and growing within you.

Your baby's so tiny, barely a speck. You probably couldn't see him with your naked eye, if you could look. Life seems hardly possible, and yet he's there, within you. He's growing so fast right now, forming germ layers and growing a skeleton. His cells are multiplying, and he's expanding.

Have you calculated your due date? Are you starting to wonder and worry about the way you'll rearrange your home and your schedule and your life?

When I'm at the very beginning of a pregnancy, I am often overwhelmed with a flurry of feelings: joy, fear, dread. Questions are suddenly everywhere, and, if I'm not careful, I'm overwhelmed with the need to make decisions about everything right now.

Pregnancy is a very physical experience, one that challenges everything you've known, even if it's not your first pregnancy. If you aren't a glowing, happy pregnant person, take heart. This is a journey with an end in sight, and the prize is another human being! We all approach pregnancy from our own perspective, and there is always room to improve our attitude and learn to be closer to God and his will for us.

I tend to be overly dramatic and focused on my physical discomforts, especially as I'm embracing the porcelain of my toilet bowl early in pregnancy. Do you find yourself complaining—even if only internally—about the hurdles? Are you struggling to keep your thoughts heavenly as your face points downward?

Walking with Mary: The Annunciation

So much of what Mary has to teach me can be found in the first Joyful Mystery, the Annunciation. When the Angel Gabriel came to Mary with the request that she be the Mother of God, she said yes.

She didn't hesitate or take a minute to think. What made her stop and ponder was the angel's greeting, not his request. She asked for clarification—"How can this be, since I have no husband?" But I can't blame her for that. It was, after all, a miracle out of all proportion with her experience.

How often do I find myself focusing on the wrong end of things and making it about me when it should be about others? How often do I ask God to give me a sign when I carry within me evidence of his mercy and love?

Being a handmaid, as Mary calls herself in her acceptance of God's request, isn't easy, but it's easier, in many ways, than saying yes without calculating the price in time, effort, and means. Letting things be done to me, as Mary did in the Annunciation and throughout her life, is a bigger challenge than struggling to control everything around me.

There are many aspects of pregnancy that you can't control. Your body will change, and you'll probably change your mind a time or two about anything and everything. You may find that you're irrational and emotional in ways you never have been before. Lean on God and reach for Mary, whose yes in the Annunciation gives you the answer to what God's asking of you.

One Small Step

There are many times when I don't think I get a lot out of Mass. It might be that the music is extra-terrible or that the priest drones on in a homily that falls flat. It might be the amount of background noise or the constant potty breaks and screams from one of my children.

If I'm honest, there are far too many times when I don't come to Mass prepared for what's going to happen. I forget to insist that the kids go potty ahead of time. I fail to feed them properly. I don't get myself in a mental state that will allow me to hear anything.

But really, the point of Mass isn't to get; I go in order to give to God: he can have my problems and my stress, my fears and my pain. In the midst of giving, I do receive: all the graces I could ever need, thanks to an hour and a miracle that's waiting for me whenever I'm willing to say yes to it.

Say yes to God this week by attending Mass with your full attention—or as much of it as your state in life will allow. As you receive the Eucharist, know that you are joined to Jesus in a special way and that he loves you.

Faith Focus

Saint Gerard Majella is the patron saint for all aspects of pregnancy. The story goes that a pregnant woman made a false accusation against him. She said he was the father of her child, and he responded with silence.[1] Ultimately his name was cleared after she retracted her statement, but his association with pregnancy remains.

Saint Gerard struggled throughout his life, first with the poverty of his upbringing and then with his desire to enter the priesthood. He was eventually ordained and even accepted into a religious order, and throughout his life, reports of miracles—and even bilocation—surrounded him.

Turning to Saint Gerard during pregnancy is natural. He has a long history of helping pregnant women, and I always imagine that he has a soft spot for expectant mothers. He's a terrific intercessor and a great friend to have in heaven.

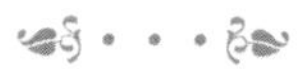

Praying Your Pregnancy

Saint Gerard, as I enter this special time of pregnancy, pray for me, that I may embrace my vocation and cherish my child. Help me to do God's will and to find peace in answering God's call. Intercede for me with God who gives all life that I may conceive and raise children to please God, in this life and in the life to come. Amen.

CHAPTER 2

Week 6 (Fetal Age: 4 Weeks)

Surprise! The Unintended Pregnancy

There are some surprises that are more pleasant than others. I find pregnancy to be, often, a love-hate sort of surprise. It's always a surprise of sorts, and while I'm thrilled (and terrified) to welcome new life, I'm often (sadly) inconvenienced.

Is there ever a good time for a baby? (Yes, I know: is there ever a bad time? Think of me what you will, but I can all too easily respond with a knee-jerk yes.)

I don't always deal well with the difference between what I have in mind and what actually happens. God and I have had many discussions (mostly one-sided) where I shake my fist and demand to know just what in the world he is thinking.

It sounds trite to say, "trust in God," and I'm the last person to be good at putting this into practice. However, when I do finally surrender my will and let even a sliver of trust in God into my approach, I find myself freed. No longer do I have to have things figured out. No more do I have the burden of knowing what comes next.

Find a friend who will listen to your rants and point you, ever-so-gently, back to God. Sit in the sun and picture the warmth of God's arms holding you, carrying you, leading you to the place he has in mind for you.

And, while it might not be medically supported or even advisable, eat some chocolate. Then pray a Hail Mary and brew some tea. Picture Mary across from you, smiling gently, and know that you'll be blessed, even if the road to it feels like a pile of rocks to climb.

NOW THAT YOU'VE BEEN PREGNANT FOR ALMOST A full month, you're probably noticing some changes. Maybe you've gained some weight, or maybe, if you can't keep things down and your appetite is poor, you have lost weight. In any event, things are different with your body.

Pregnancy is not an illness, though at this point it can feel like one. When I'm hugging the toilet and cradling my head to avoid any further outburst, I have a hard time remembering that the child within me is a blessing. When I find myself considering all that's wrong with the world and the many dangers of life, I can get myself into a funk of wondering why we bother to have children. It is so easy to forget the hope I feel when I see a baby's unconditional gaze, the peace I feel when I ponder her tiny perfection, and the fulfillment she brings to the world through her very life.

There is a price to blessings, and, for me, that price is one of trust. I have to trust that God knows what's best and that he can bring great good from whatever situation I find myself in. I have to trust that the temporal discomfort—the puking, the heartburn, and the loss of appetite—will give way to a greater good.

During this week, your baby's heart tubes fuse, and her heart contractions begin.[2] She already has a beating heart, even though she's tiny. If you have an ultrasound during this week or any time thereafter, you'll probably see the heartbeats.

Every beat of that little heart is proof of God's love. It seems impossible. Conception is unlikely enough, but the growing baby is even more shocking. There are so many vulnerabilities that an embryo faces in the first developmental stage: how she makes it all the way to birth is really quite a miracle.

In the tiny thump-thump of my baby's heartbeat, I have so often felt the assurance of God. I never wanted children of my own. I never saw motherhood as a goal of any kind. God didn't let that stop the miracle from occurring though. As I continue through my journey of motherhood, facing the overwhelming task of caring for souls, I think back to the first few weeks of pregnancy with a combination of dread and wonder. A beating heart within me seems, somehow, to make the discomfort more worthwhile. It makes what's happening to my life real in a way that changes the entire world: there is another person, another soul, now alive.

Walking with Mary: The Visitation

Mary was in these early days of pregnancy when she made the long journey to visit her cousin Elizabeth. Was her trip punctuated with potty stops? Did she find herself wishing for her own bed during the days she spent getting there?

However miserable Mary might have felt in her first trimester, she didn't hesitate to serve. She knew Elizabeth, who was elderly, must need help. Beyond that, she provided an encouragement to her cousin that was probably worth far more than any of the cleaning or cooking she did during her three months in Judea.

Serving isn't easy when you don't feel well. It's hard enough when you're busy with your own life and juggling your own obligations, but insert physical hardships—even if it's just not feeling 100 percent—and it becomes a huge hurdle. It takes extra effort to serve in any capacity, and that's what Mary shows us.

She might have been throwing up every few hours, unable to keep anything down, without a taste for anything. She might have just longed for a nap. Elizabeth probably knew this and more than likely encouraged Mary to rest. But I don't think Mary made the arduous journey there and back only to let Elizabeth coddle her. I picture her reproaching Elizabeth for trying to do too much. It was Mary taking over the household duties.

In Mary's embrace of Elizabeth, I find an example of serving when I least want to, of expending extra effort for others, and of giving in the most generous way. She gave, and in giving to Elizabeth, she also gave to each of us. She shows us, quietly and without fanfare, what it is to joyously accept our vocation. Her joy overflowed in the Magnificat, despite discomfort and uncertainty.

Our joy can overflow too, no matter what hurdles we face. Maybe, like Mary, what we need to do is give ourselves to another in service.

One Small Step

I have a confession to make: I fear pregnancy. It's not so much the discomfort or the way labor and delivery looms before me. I fear for my baby in many ways, and for my family should we face an infant loss or miscarriage. One sure way I've found to battle my fears (and, incidentally, my physical discomforts) is to be of service to others. It helps me to keep my mind off the fear of unexpected—and unpleasant—surprises.

Our parish has offered a Eucharistic Adoration program for a number of years, and spending time with Jesus, one-on-one, always soothes my frantic fears. I find that praying for others—there's never a shortage of people who have bigger prayer requests than I do—and giving some of my time to Jesus to be the best balm.

If you aren't well enough to make it to church to pray before Jesus in the Blessed Sacrament, you could also spend time in prayer at home or offering your pregnancy-related challenges and struggles in communion with others who are suffering throughout the world and in your parish family.

The most important work we do is that which unites us to God more fully and completely, though that work is often simple and unremarkable. It includes thankless tasks, smiling through pain, and even accepting where we are and what God has in store for us.

Give Jesus your fears, and ask him to help you serve the people in your life this week. Ask your Creator to hold you close during your pregnancy. Pray for your baby and your family. Allow yourself to be cradled in God's arms and listen for the whispering encouragement he sends to you.

Faith Focus

"But he said to me, 'My grace is sufficient for you, for power is made perfect in weakness.' I will rather boast most gladly of my weaknesses, in order that the power of Christ may dwell with me" (2 Cor 12:9).

I rarely feel as weak as I do when I'm pregnant. Read this verse this week—maybe even post it somewhere you will see it often—and feel the comfort of God's grace at work in your body.

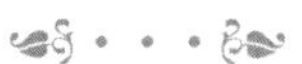

Praying Your Pregnancy

Lord, through your Blessed Mother, you give me an example of how to serve others even in the midst of the discomfort of these early weeks of pregnancy. Help me to follow in her footsteps and, like Elizabeth, rejoice in the presence of your son every step of the way. Guide me to the comfort of your presence, and hold me in any worries I harbor. Amen.

CHAPTER 3

Week 7
(Fetal Age: 5 Weeks)

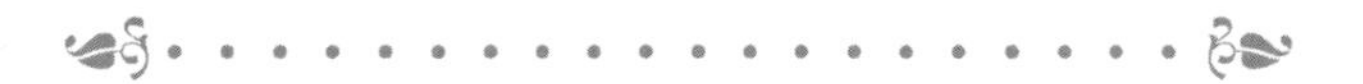

Eating Disorders during Pregnancy

By Kate Wicker

During my first pregnancy, it was awe inspiring to reflect upon the mystery of new life and how my body was capable of growing another human being, and even more amazingly, was providing sanctuary to a new soul with eternal value.

My newfound appreciation for my body unfortunately did not carry through during the early postpartum period or during my subsequent pregnancies. I found it very difficult to watch the numbers on the scale increase or to feel my clothing fit tighter and tighter.

I finally realized I needed to stop stepping on the scale or at least not know the exact number because it was starting to resurrect the old demons that told me my worth was found in my ability to weigh a certain number and the erroneous belief that I was powerful because I was able to whip my body into submission. I was blessed to have an amazing Catholic midwife with whom I openly shared my struggles. She helped me not make my weight an issue and did not force me to have regular weigh-ins.

Shunning the scale for a woman with an eating-disorder history can be very liberating.

If you've struggled with an eating disorder in the past, I encourage you to be up front with your health-care provider. The health-care provider needs to know that it may be difficult for you to watch your body change and gain weight sometimes at an alarming rate! Not all medical professionals understand the dynamics of your eating disorder (too many people assume it's just about being thin when the destructive habits—purging by using laxatives or inducing vomiting, starving, exercising compulsively, or binge eating—are vehicles for expressing much deeper issues). You may want to hand the health-care provider a letter in which you explain how your eating disorder evolved, what triggered it, and what has helped you heal.

There are some health-care providers who are very vigilant about weight gain during pregnancy. While I understand they have the concern of the mom and baby's health in mind, this approach would have been damaging to me because I was already hyperaware of the changes my body was going through.

If you find yourself pregnant before you have overcome some of your disordered eating, it's imperative you're up front about your struggles. Restricting calories, purging with self-induced vomiting or laxatives, and/or binge eating can also be harmful to your own body as well as your developing baby. With courage, God's grace, the help of a compassionate health-care provider, therapy, and/or other clinical treatment, you can work to adopt more healthful habits to help ensure a healthy baby.

Even women who have never struggled with a clinical eating disorder may find the physical changes of pregnancy difficult to handle. When faced with feeling less than beautiful, remind yourself that gaining weight and any other physical changes you may have to endure during pregnancy are due to the incredible miracle unfolding within you. Do your best to eat well. Treat your body with respect. Exercise if you have the green light from your provider, and you'll likely gain the amount of weight needed to nurture a healthy baby.

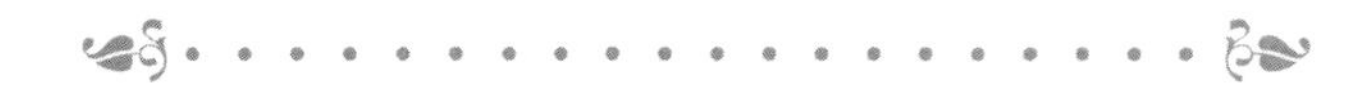

YOUR BABY IS THE SIZE OF A BB PELLET, AND YOU'RE probably marveling that someone so small can make such a big impact. This is a big week for growth, and your little one will be doubling in size.[3]

Have you struggled with heartburn and constipation? Are you hugging a toilet and wondering when the sun will shine on you again? Do your clothes fit awkwardly; does your food taste slightly off and your body long for sleep at every hour?

Maybe pregnancy is novel, and the hardships aren't a big deal to you, or maybe you find yourself facing a mountain of dislikes and discomforts. We all have a slightly different approach to pregnancy, and I always find myself feeling guilty for any negative feelings I have. After observing the infertility struggles of many in my life and seeing babies buried, I always feel very unworthy of pregnancy. So many families would welcome a baby heartily while I do so begrudgingly at best!

There's a power to pregnancy that seems to affect people in a way they just can't help. You'll hear the word "miracle" from people who aren't religious. You'll see a gentleness from those who claim never to have wanted children. Your pregnancy is proof of how we are made and designed by God: within you is new life.

On the other hand, you may notice the opposite. It's too early for you to be able to proclaim your pregnancy with your appearance, but pregnancy will probably come up in conversation, either casually or intentionally, and then you may find yourself the recipient of all that helpful advice—and the horror stories of labor.

Before you give in to the despair, worry, and hilarity that are sure to ensue, pause and turn your mind to God. Ask Mama Mary to hold your hand and protect you from the mental hijacking that can so easily occur when well-meaning people start to share more than you care to hear. Remember the joy of new life, and find a reason to smile this week, no matter how negative you're tempted to feel. Your feelings, while in many ways uncontrollable, are also not reality or the lens through which you have to view the world—and this pregnancy.

Walking with Mary: The Nativity

In the Nativity, Mary gave birth to the Savior of the world, Jesus Christ. Animals surrounded her, and Joseph was probably feeling more than a little unsure of himself. On that first Christmas, in the most unlikely and humble surroundings, the long-awaited Messiah was born.

My first reaction to reflection on the Nativity is usually something to the effect of, "Poor Mary! A cold cave, a bunch of rag-tag visitors right away, and no heated blankets!" My priorities are obviously much different from Mary's, and maybe that's why I find this mystery so fruitful for meditation in my twenty-first-century, first-world life.

When I'm holding a new baby of my own with all the comforts available to me, praying this mystery can seem light-years away from where I am. Jesus was born into poverty, and his life started in a cave in Bethlehem, far from his parents' home. Though kings visited him, the first real welcoming committee was a group of simple shepherds, who must have brought a pretty strong aroma with them.

Somehow, I doubt Mary minded. New moms love to share their babies, and she had a pretty special baby to share.

All the same, as rich as I am—in stuff but also in distraction—I wonder if I shouldn't seek that simplicity of the Nativity more often. Much of the preparation for a baby involves stuff—diapers and blankets, socks and Onesies, and bedding and toys. It's amazing how much a tiny little person requires, but we have a tendency to go overboard too.

In the Nativity, we see the importance of not concentrating so much on the material things. Just as Mary and Joseph trusted God to provide, we need to lean into our heavenly Father and allow him to give us what we need. As your body expands with the new life inside you, so your soul can expand to welcome God's love and care, but only if you remove the attachment you may have to the material.

One Small Step

It's so easy to imagine all that can go wrong during pregnancy. It's amazing, in fact, that life continues, babies are born, and mothers survive.

All that, though, feeds my worry during pregnancy. Something about the hormones feeds my natural obsessive tendencies, and I always struggle with fear of "losing" my baby (though I know no baby is ever truly "mine").

A few years before my husband and I were married, when we were dating and I was a newly minted Catholic, his sister lost a baby as a full-term stillborn. I was the person who took my future mother-in-law to the funeral home; I watched the family pull together and grieve. More than anything, I was impacted by the knowledge that the small white casket at the front of the chapel was filled with hope.

I had never seen a casket so small; I had never witnessed a grief like the loss of a baby before. In the many years since, I have seen how my sister-in-law has allowed that apparent tragedy to be, instead, a beacon of hope to those around her. Instead of holding it close to herself and letting it make her bitter, she has shared it and helped others.

Even so, I struggle when I'm pregnant, and I have a hard time being around certain people too much. I feel their worry as my burden—and I've come to realize that I may only be imagining things! I may be projecting my own terror of burying a baby, my own concerns about what could happen, and my own thoughts on how things might unravel.

One help that I've found is to have my priest bless me during my pregnancy. It's a humbling experience—much like having your feet washed during Holy Thursday Mass, if you ever have that opportunity—and it's a lot like asking for help. And actually, it is help, help of the very best kind: divine!

At this point, your priest may not even know you are pregnant, but he will probably be happy to bless you—and specifically your belly if you are comfortable with that. It might be hard to ask, but I encourage you to swallow whatever pride or hesitation is blocking your reception of the graces that a blessing will bring.

Your priest may choose to use the Rite of Blessing for a Child in the Womb. The rite happens to contain a beautiful prayer that you can pray at home:

God, author of all life,
bless, we pray, this unborn child,
give constant protection
and grant a healthy birth
that is the sign of our rebirth one day
into the eternal rejoicing of heaven. . . .

—excerpt from the Prayer of Blessing

Faith Focus

In the *Catechism of the Catholic Church*, we read, "Illness can lead to anguish, self-absorption, sometimes even despair and revolt against God. It can also make a person more mature, helping him discern in his life what is not essential so that he can turn toward that which is. Very often illness provokes a search for God and a return to him" (1499).

If you were to substitute "pregnancy" for "illness" in the previous paragraph, you would learn very quickly how I tend to view pregnancy. Thankfully, pregnancy is not an illness after all. No matter how I may feel each time I find myself sick or exhausted, the child growing inside of me is God's plan for life; it's not an illness.

This section of the *Catechism* deals with Anointing of the Sick, a sacrament that many people have not taken advantage of. You don't need to be dying to receive it and request it. "The Anointing of the Sick 'is not a sacrament for those only who are at the point of death. Hence, as soon as anyone of the faithful begins to be in danger from sickness or old age, the fitting time for him to receive this sacrament has certainly already arrived'" (1514).

Whether you're struggling with a chronic condition in your pregnancy or something pops up that worries you, don't hesitate to request this sacrament. It involves a priest or bishop praying over you and then anointing you with blessed oil. You receive great graces from anointing, including strength, peace, and courage to overcome (1520), union with Jesus's passion (1521), and the intercession of the saints praying for you in heaven (1522).

Praying Your Pregnancy

Lord, there's so much that could go wrong and that might go wrong. Free me from the overwhelming burden of my worries and my fears. Hold me close to you, and give me the courage to accept the graces I need for this journey through pregnancy. Pave the way ahead of me with your love, and guide me to fulfilling your will. Amen.

CHAPTER 4

Week 8 (Fetal Age: 6 Weeks)

When Do You Tell?

One question that always comes up with every pregnancy is how and when to make the announcement. On the one hand, there's the line of thinking that advises pregnant couples to wait to tell anyone until they are safely in the second trimester, past the highest risks of miscarriage. On the other hand, the excitement of finding out that there will be a new a member in a family is too much to keep quiet, and I find that this is the approach that works best for us.

For one thing, my biggest support during pregnancy is the group of people whom I always want to tell first. Those family members and friends pray for me, first of all, and they also understand why I'm suddenly more of a monster to be around.

Secondly, in the event of a miscarriage, I want to be able to share my pain with people who will care about it as much as I do. I want my current children to remind me of the joy ahead even as I'm doubled over the toilet or feeling like a hormonal tornado.

When you tell—and whom you tell—is something you and your husband have to discern. My husband and I always tell our parents before we tell anyone else.

You might hesitate to tell some people because you know they'll have a negative reaction. You might not want to have to explain the sad news in the event of a high-risk pregnancy.

Surround yourself with prayer warriors, and tell your good news when—and to whom—you discern it will be best.

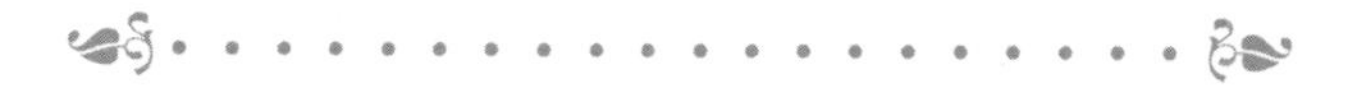

YOUR BABY IS GROWING AND IS NOW ABOUT THE SIZE of a pinto bean.[4] His ears are forming both internally and externally. By now he has elbows and the beginnings of fingers and toes (called digital and toe rays).[5]

It's the second month of your journey through pregnancy, and it's probably still new to you. Maybe you haven't even told anyone that you're pregnant. You may still be wearing regular clothes, though they're probably tighter on you.

You may be experiencing some aches and pains, and you may even be starting to have some sciatic nerve pain. Your skin might be changing, and when you look in the mirror, you might have a flashback to the acne of your junior-high days.

At about this point in pregnancy, I always feel torn, like there's an impossible amount of time ahead of me, but yet as though, knowing how time flies, there's not at all enough time to prepare. There always seems to be a list of preparations that's daunting, involves help from others, and requires tools, knowledge, and planning.

Few things take over your life like a pregnancy, and I always feel guilty when I hate it: so many people I know long for children, so many women I know have struggled with losses, and so many children are aborted each year. Surely I can embrace the joy and ignore the discomfort, right?

If you find yourself moody and miserable, I encourage you to turn to God in prayer. Give it to him, and lay it on him. He can handle it, and he's happy that you came to him with your problems. Put your head in his lap, let his arms encircle you, and let go of the things that weigh on you right now, from family to work to your physical state.

If you're bursting with joy, share it. Is there someone who can benefit from a smile, your sunny disposition, or a jolt of hope in a world full of negativity? Can you encourage someone else in a way that brings light to the world?

Walking with Mary: The Presentation

It took me a while to relate to Mary and Joseph's actions in the Presentation as acts of obedience. Obedience isn't something I naturally relate to—one of my greatest weaknesses is accepting authority. During my journey to and in the Catholic Church, once I understood that there is a higher authority than me, I found myself free in a way I had never been before.

Mary and Joseph didn't go to the Temple with the baby Jesus just because it was what people did: they did it out of obedience. When Mary heard Simeon's prophecy and then his conclusion that a sword would pierce her heart (see Lk 2:34–35), what must she have thought? What went through her mind, or did she save it for later because she didn't know what to think?

In my own life, I've heard God's voice plenty of times from the mouths of others. It's uncanny, no matter how many times it happens to me. When a child or a friend looks at me and says something that is like a thought of mine come to life, I can't help but shake my head. How could he or she have known what was on my heart, when I hadn't told anyone? It is proof, so often, of God at work in the very interior of my life. Who else knows—or even cares about—my very deepest desires and my unimportant-to-anyone-else's thoughts?

I suspect that God has to use the people around me because I'll ignore or discount that still small voice that will whisper in my mind. I'll question it until I'm convinced it's nothing.

That is the time he uses the people around me to help me understand.

Mary was far more in touch with the Spirit than I am, and I look to her for guidance. In the Presentation, she models listening to what someone else says and respecting it as important, without knowing what it means exactly. What Simeon told Mary ("and you yourself a sword will pierce," [Lk 2:35]) was difficult. It wasn't easy to understand. It didn't sound really promising—who wants to have a sword pierce her, after all? And yet, Mary says yes. She embraces her role, once again. She obeys. She listens and respects and gives me yet another reason to ponder her as an example for my own life.

One Small Step

Do you remember your Baptism? My own Baptism, as an adult, differed a great deal from what I experienced with my children as infants. At Easter Masses we are called upon to renew our Baptismal promises, but we can do it on a personal level at any time.

This week, make it a point to go to church and pray in front of the Blessed Sacrament. Renew the promises that you made with your Baptism (or that your parents made for you, if you were an infant or young child). Try starting with this prayer from Saint Louis de Montfort:

> I, who through the tender mercy of the Eternal Father was privileged to be baptized "in the name of the Lord Jesus" (Acts 19:5) and thus to share in the dignity of his divine Sonship, wish now in the presence of this same loving Father and of his only-begotten Son to renew in all sincerity the promises I solemnly made at the time of my holy Baptism. I, therefore, now do once again renounce Satan; I renounce all his works; I renounce all his allurements. I believe in God, the Father almighty, Creator of heaven and earth. I believe in Jesus Christ, his only Son, our Lord, who was born into this world and who suffered and died for my sins and rose again. I believe in the Holy Spirit, the Holy Catholic Church, the

> communion of Saints, the forgiveness of sins, the resurrection of the body and life everlasting. Having been buried with Christ unto death and raised up with him unto a new life, I promise to live no longer for myself or for that world which is the enemy of God but for him who died for me and rose again, serving God, my heavenly Father, faithfully and unto death in the holy Catholic Church. Taught by our Savior's command and formed by the word of God, I now dare to say: Our Father, who art in heaven, hallowed be thy name; thy kingdom come; thy will be done on earth as it is in heaven. Give us this day our daily bread; and forgive us our trespasses as we forgive those who trespass against us; and lead us not into temptation, but deliver us from evil. Amen.[6]

Faith Focus

Novenas are a wonderful way to pray for a specific intention. Traditionally, they involve nine periods of prayer (usually days, though some are hours or weeks or even months) and come in many different formats and with any intention you could imagine.

Pregnancy is naturally a period of turning to God, and its length—nine months—lends itself to a novena. Spend the next nine days praying for your family—including your in-utero baby.

Find a prayer you like and pray it for nine days to gain a sense of the pattern, rhythm, and timing. Then do some research and find a dedicated novena that strikes a chord with you. Imagine yourself walking up to Jesus, just as Mary and Joseph met Simeon in the Temple at the Presentation. Turn your pregnancy—including your hopes and dreams, fears and anxieties—over to God while you pray during the length of your novena.

Praying Your Pregnancy

This is all so new to me, God, and I can't help but marvel at how you, too, were as small and vulnerable as my baby is right now. Your mother, too, experienced the aches and pains of pregnancy. Let me turn to her this week and use her example to remind me of the joys of obedience. Amen.

CHAPTER 5

Week 9 (Fetal Age: 7 Weeks)

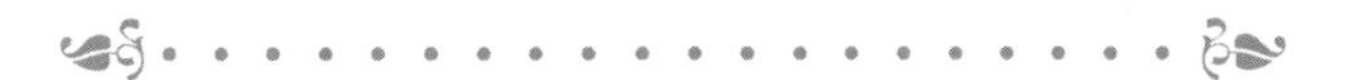

Miscarriage

By Mary DeTurris Poust

Every year, as August 6 nears, I feel myself moving inward a bit, toward a quiet place deep inside reserved for the baby I call Grace, my second baby, the baby I never got to hold.

With a mother's intuition, I had known something was wrong during that pregnancy. When you are a mother, you just seem to know things about your children, even when there is no logical reason you should, even when they are still growing inside you. With that same mother's intuition, no matter how busy or stressed I am, no matter how many things I seem to forget as I drive my other three children to and fro, I never forget the anniversary of my miscarriage. It is imprinted on my heart.

Although the powerful initial grief has faded with each passing year, my love for Grace and my connection to her never fade because over time I have come to recognize Grace's great gift to us. She has shaped our family by her absence rather than her presence.

I am very much aware of the fact that life would be very different had she lived. She managed to leave her mark on us, even without taking a breath. She lingers here, not only in my heart but also around the edges of our lives—especially the lives of our two girls who followed her. I know them because I did not know Grace. What a sorrowful and beautiful impact she has had.

Women who have suffered through a miscarriage know what it means to have an empty space in our soul, to cry out to God in anguish for a little life lost too soon. But if we have faith and if we continue to celebrate that unborn life year after year, we emerge from our grief filled with gratitude for the way our baby has left an imprint on this world without ever setting foot on earth.

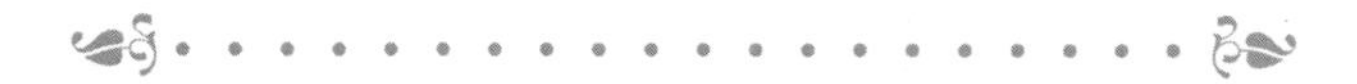

YOUR BABY HAS FINGERS AND TOES NOW. SHE'S squirming around inside of you, though you probably can't feel movement yet. In the few weeks of her life, your baby has gone from a person comprised of just a few cells to a person who's moving and active. What's even more amazing is that you might not have even known for sure that you were pregnant before this point!

Those little hands, flexed inside your uterus, are more than a mere developmental milestone for you and your baby. They are a reminder of the adventure you are about to begin. These very hands will beg for your embrace and resist your attempts to keep them clean. Those same little fingers will find their way into every mess imaginable one day. Her palms will bear the markings of finger paint as she creates your most treasured work of art. At some point, she will pick up a pencil and write you a letter, or a poem. She may even help you clean the house or do the dishes with these hands that are fully formed inside of you.

God willing, you will some day see these fingers laced together in prayer to Jesus. And before you know it, these same hands that are currently smaller than a nickel will be turning the keys in the ignition of a car and leading your child to places beyond your reach. Ultimately, the development of your baby's hands is the perfect reminder to turn your gaze heavenward as you reflect on what's happening inside of you because these are the same hands that will hold the strings to your heart.

Walking with Mary: Finding Jesus in the Temple

I had a few years of enjoying young children in the form of younger siblings and nieces and nephews before I was married and started having my own. I thought I was ready for the reality of children saying the darndest things.

Nothing, though, could have prepared me for the hilarity—and heartbreak—I have experienced as a mom. From my children's mouths I've heard tender expressions of love but also explosions of anger. They've made observations that have lifted my spirits and others that have cut me to the quick.

When Mary and Joseph find Jesus after three days of searching for him (see Lk 2:42–51), they must have had some heat in their words to him. Maybe I'm projecting a bit, but maybe worry is, to some extent, a natural reaction of parents to the experience of losing a child in a crowd or a store.

What I learn from this mystery is how the story continues with him going home and being obedient, even in the face of what seems to be a smart-aleck remark from Jesus—"Didn't you know where I'd be?" This seems like it would be a prime time to uphold parental authority, but in the silence, I find a lesson in humility.

Just as your baby would be hard to find right now—she's about as big as a green olive[7]—still, she is there. Jesus was in the Temple all along, though his parents didn't know it and had to search for him. Their inability to find him didn't change where he was the entire time.

In the Temple, Jesus was listening and asking questions much like a typical twelve-year-old. Yet he was anything but typical. I find comfort, though, in the idea that he wasn't born with all the knowledge he needed. In this way, his humanity is expressed in this mystery, as is the quandary of his parents: do they punish him after this or are they so glad to find him that they just let him off the hook?

In this mystery, we can find ourselves at Jesus's feet, asking for the guidance to be the kind of parent he's calling us to be. Though it's early in the journey of parenting this particular child, we don't have to wait to ask to be able to cooperate with the graces God sends our way in our parenting journey.

One Small Step

Jesus gives us an example in the mystery of the Finding in the Temple: he's in his Father's house. God is our Father too, and we find ourselves in his house at least once a week.

Taking a lesson from Jesus, spend the week reading and reflecting on the scripture readings for the upcoming weekend Mass. Allow ten minutes every day to read and pray with them. You might find that on Sunday your experience of hearing the Word of God during Mass is changed and enhanced.

Faith Focus

How often do you read the Bible? You are probably exposed to it more than you give yourself credit for—Mass isn't just steeped in direct quotes from the Bible, but the entire tradition and flow of the Mass comes straight out of scripture.

If you make time every day to read the daily Mass readings, using a resource such as the *Magnificat* magazine, an app on your smartphone or device, or one of the many websites available, you'll read most of the Bible in a three-year period. The benefit of reading the Bible this way is that the connections between old covenant and new covenant are made by the choice of readings: you see prophecies fulfilled when, for example, the Old Testament reading is from Isaiah and the gospel shows how it's fulfilled.

Praying Your Pregnancy

Give me the courage to turn to your word, Lord, and let it be a lamp lighting my way through the dark times I may experience during pregnancy. Help me to find your son, and guide me as I search for him in my day and through my sufferings, however large or small they are. Amen.

CHAPTER 6

Week 10 (Fetal Age: 8 Weeks)

THIS WEEK, YOUR BABY DEFINITELY LOOKS MORE human and can now be weighed, because he is big enough.[8] He's the size of a small plum and is now, officially, no longer an embryo; he is a full-fledged fetus![9] All of his organs are now formed.[10]

You might feel like a completely different person—your breasts are likely sore and tender, various parts of your body might take turns crying out in pain, and you may be riding an emotional roller-coaster unlike any you've ridden before.

What if it's not going the way you planned or envisioned? Are you finding that pregnancy is an unwelcome surprise? Do you wonder how any good can come from it?

Years ago, before I had any notions of being married, much less of being a mother, a colleague of mine often trumpeted, "Feelings are not reality." I chuckle now, because, though I consider myself a highly rational member of the female gender, I'm still a woman, and my hormones get the best of me more often than I'd like, especially during pregnancy.

I never think of the fact that my husband's life is changing, just as mine is. He might not be carrying the baby inside him, but he has to deal with a whole host of considerations. In my discussions with my husband as I was preparing this manuscript, I asked him about his concerns during the period of time when I'm pregnant. I expected to hear all about finances and responsibility, but I quickly learned that his questions and fears were just as grave as mine. He immediately peppered me with hypothetical questions like, "What if the baby dies during pregnancy or childbirth? What will I do if you die during childbirth? How can I raise a family without you? Who will teach the girls all the things I don't know about? With my age being a factor, who will be there for them when I do pass if I were to lose you? Who will see them graduate high school or college? Who will guide them on their way through life?"

As the tears blurred my eyes during our discussion, he raised the point that I couldn't have raised on my own. "Losing a baby would be tragic, but my biggest fear would be losing you. I never worried about money or material things."

My husband's background prepares him for fatherhood each time, uniquely and perhaps differently than your husband's background. My husband was raised poor and saw, firsthand, God provide. In the time before we were married, his two sisters buried three full-term babies between them.

His stark admission of his fears—at a time when we were not facing pregnancy—made me realize how very different we are in our approach. With past pregnancies I faced a million worries and fears, and I never asked him what he worried about. Honestly, I didn't think I could handle it at the time. I'm glad to know now, though, and I will hold his fears close to my heart and in my prayers if and when we are blessed with another pregnancy.

Consider talking to your husband about his fears (and yours). You may learn something new about each other. Or, it may turn into a "moment of truth" when you find yourselves talking about all kinds of things regarding your married and family life. Ask Jesus to take part, too, by beginning with a prayer for openness and honest communication in your marriage. You might find that he has something to add to the conversation.

Walking with Mary: The Baptism of Jesus

Jesus didn't need to be baptized, and John the Baptist didn't waste any time pointing that out to him. Even so, when Jesus insisted, John obeyed and baptized Jesus.

In this way, Jesus united himself to each of us who is baptized. I imagine that, just as my son is the spitting image of my husband and my daughter looks exactly like my sister-in-law, Baptism makes us look more like Christ.

Who better to resemble than him? Although it's not an easy path he chose, filled with poverty, suffering, and rejection, he also brought joy to the whole world through his many miracles and healings.

Both of my daughters are "daddy's girls" and it always makes me smile to see him melt as they clamor for his attention. I remember being a "daddy's girl" many years ago. I hope that now, using Jesus's example, I can be a different kind of daddy's girl, one who is never far from my heavenly daddy and who climbs into his lap with gusto and confidence.

Hold your arms up, and let your heavenly daddy embrace you, whether you're scared or hurt, confused or bitter. Be a daddy's girl of the very best kind, and strive to hear him say to you, as he said to Jesus, "You are my beloved Son; with you I am well pleased" (Mk 1:11).

One Small Step

I remember the first time I ventured to the front of our small church and lit a votive candle. I wasn't sure what to do, but I did what I'd seen everyone else do: I slipped my money in the box, knelt down, and lit a candle. I looked up at the statue of Mary and asked her to help me with my special intention.

Over the years, I've become more comfortable with this, and I've even been known to light a candle when I notice that there aren't any lit. As my mother-in-law once said, "We can't let the prayers go out!" Though I know people are still praying, I love the visual of a lit candle, and sometimes I'll even light candles in my own home as a reminder to pray throughout the day.

This week, light a candle at your church. There is no special power in the candle itself. You make a personal sacrifice to donate money for the candle. The candle "carries" your prayers to heaven as it continues to burn after you leave. It imprints itself as a bright spot on your mind. Let that bright spot be the point you turn to this week, seeking God's providence in all that you do.

Faith Focus

Confirmation and Baptism are two of the sacraments of initiation. Through them, we have the foundations of our lives as Christians. The *Catechism* explains it in detail in paragraph 1212:

> The sacraments of Christian initiation—Baptism, Confirmation, and the Eucharist—lay the foundations of every Christian life. "The sharing in the divine nature given to men through the grace of Christ bears a certain likeness to the origin, development, and nourishing of natural life. The faithful are born anew by Baptism, strengthened by the sacrament of Confirmation, and receive in the Eucharist the food of eternal life. By means of these sacraments of Christian initiation, they thus receive in increasing measure the treasures of the divine life and advance toward the perfection of charity.

In Confirmation, we receive the seven gifts of the Holy Spirit: fear of the Lord, piety, knowledge, understanding, counsel, wisdom, and fortitude. We are marked with the seal of the Holy Spirit, which can never be removed or replaced.

At your Baptism, the paschal candle was lit, and you or your parents received a candle as a symbol of the light of Christ. It is a reminder to follow the path of Christ. In his own Baptism, Jesus was unveiled as the Son of God. After his Baptism, there was no turning back: His way was forward to Calvary. No matter how you may stray or make mistakes in your life, thanks to the sacrament of Confirmation, you belong to Christ and are protected by him. Here's what the *Catechism* says in paragraph 1296:

> Christ himself declared that he was marked with his Father's seal. Christians are also marked with a seal: "It is God who establishes us with you in Christ and has

commissioned us; he has put his seal on us and given us his Spirit in our hearts as a guarantee." This seal of the Holy Spirit marks our total belonging to Christ, our enrollment in his service forever, as well as the promise of divine protection in the great eschatological trial.

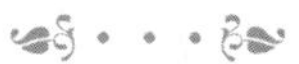

Praying Your Pregnancy

It's quite a ride, Lord, being pregnant, and it's hard to look at you and expect you to understand. You were never pregnant! I know, though, that you must somehow understand my trials and that you care. When I doubt that, give me the strength to turn to your Mother, who surely had at least some of the troubles I do. Give me compassion for those around me, even though I'm facing my own problems; and help me, in some small way, to represent your love to them. Amen.

CHAPTER 7

Week 11 (Fetal Age: 9 Weeks)

PICK UP A LARGE LIME, AND YOU'LL HAVE AN IDEA OF how big your baby is this week.[11] It's almost the end of your first trimester, and your baby will be doing some major growing in the coming weeks.

Among the many changes taking place, this is the week your baby grows her first set of fingernails. Think of painting those little nails someday or picking the dirt out from under them. What will the little hands attached to those tiny fingernails do? How much building, playing, and moving?

I've never been able to grow fingernails with much success, except during pregnancy. It was a wonderful side effect of pregnancy, though I caught myself forgetting to make much of it since I don't normally do much with my nails (except bite them).

One of my daughters was born with what looked like a French manicure, her small fingers perfectly posed and the fingernails shaped perfectly, bright white on the ends. When I was admiring the hands and feet of my other two newborns, I couldn't help but notice how differently they were shaped than mine.

Our hands do so much in the course of our lives. They hold others and prepare meals. They type e-mails and texts and hold the pens with which we write lists and notes. They stroke fevered foreheads and clasp a loved one's shoulder. They pick and prod and poke. Over time, they show our age and our background. They become callused as a testament to our years of labor, service, and caring for others.

At only nine weeks old, the baby inside you has fingernails. She is a marvel of tiny workmanship, and your role in her life is only beginning. As her external genitalia form and become distinguished this week and become more distinct in the coming weeks, you may know with some certainty whether her hands will play with dolls or monster trucks (or both, if your children are anything like mine).

At my wedding, one of our friends took a close-up of our hands intertwined as we walked out of the church. When I look back on that day, the beginning of my vocation as a wife, I think of that picture and how solidly we were holding hands. When I look from our wedding day to now, I see that picture representing how we have to rely on each other, almost to the point of forgetting where one of us ends and the other begins.

Pregnancy is a mystery that unveils itself slowly into a new person. As you host that little person within you, hold hands with Mary, our mother. Let her guide you, one baby step at a time, closer to the baby she nurtured and raised. Feel the confidence and peace that can only come from resting in God's care.

Walking with Mary: The Wedding at Cana

She looks around and sees a celebration, the union of two people at the beginning of their life together. It is the ending of each as individuals and the start of the two as one.

It's just like a mother to stick her nose in to try to fix things, isn't it? I never understood this tendency until my oldest daughter was whisked away in an ambulance one night with stroke-like symptoms. My husband rode with her, and I followed after finding someone to watch our other daughter.

I just wanted things fixed, but there was no one nearby. I called a close friend and her first suggestion was to call on Mary for help. As she led me in prayer, I felt a wellspring of something, and I think now that it was hope. I had no idea what was going to happen with my five-year-old, I didn't know what the future held, and I couldn't do a thing about it except pray and accept God's will.

It seems a stretch to compare this to the wedding at Cana, but to that couple, the crisis they were facing was every bit as real as what my husband and I faced with our child in an ambulance that winter night. The couple was going to suffer extreme shame in their culture, and it would have been a terrible start to their life together.

Mary did what mothers do, and she fixed things. Unlike the rest of us, who often can only offer a word of comfort or a prayer of petition, she was able to get Jesus directly involved. Come to think of it, she still plays that role, and we would do well to remember that when we pray this mystery of the Rosary.

Just as she jumped in to help a young couple at their wedding feast, so she will jump in to help the rest of us when we ask (and sometimes when we don't). She has the most direct line to God. Her only request was her instructions for the steward, "Do whatever he tells you."

My husband I had to lean on each other that winter night and in the years since. Parenthood and marriage combine to make us stronger in our weaknesses. We remind each other of the need to turn to God and rely only on his will; we hold each other when we fall and lift each other toward the One who will be our ultimate comfort.

One Small Step

Marriage is the only sacrament in which the people receiving the sacrament are also the ministers of the sacrament (*CCC*, 1623). Because it's a sacrament, marriage grants both spouses special grace, with Christ as the source (*CCC*, 1641–42). The *Catechism* expresses it beautifully: "Christ dwells with them, gives them the strength to take up their crosses and so follow him, to rise again after they have fallen, to forgive one another, to bear one another's burdens, to 'be subject to one another out of reverence for Christ,' and to love one another with supernatural, tender, and fruitful love. In the joys of their love and family life he gives them here on earth a foretaste of the wedding feast of the Lamb" (1642).

Nothing has so tested my marriage like becoming a parent. I have caught myself questioning my husband's thoughts and decisions. I've also seen myself totally ignore him in order to be "Mom."

There's no helping the overlap of roles, and, truthfully, I love my husband more deeply now that we're sharing this adventure and challenge of parenthood than I did back when we were just dating. We are a team now, but it's a harder game. There are more players, and the playing field is never the same for very long. We need the graces of the sacrament of marriage every single day.

This week, plan a special date with your spouse, and make it happen. Then take an evening or two. With a notebook, a box of envelopes, and an idea of what you enjoy doing together, write down twelve ideas of things you can do together at home. Once your baby's born, pull these envelopes out and have a date night every month.

Begin a habit that will make you the best parent you can be. Continue dating your spouse, and tap into the graces of your marriage.

Faith Focus

Jesus's first public sign was at a wedding, because his mom asked him. I take this as a sign of the importance of marriage. Jesus is present in my marriage, just as he was present there, which makes my marriage—despite the difficult days and challenging times—good in the best sense of the word.

In 1981, Blessed John Paul II released the apostolic exhortation, *Familiaris Consortio* (On the Role of the Christian Family in the Modern World). In it, he outlined what the nature and tasks of a Christian family are. He references families as "domestic churches" and challenges us to build up families as we can.[12]

> The family finds in the plan of God the Creator and Redeemer not only its identity, what it is, but also its

mission, what it can and should do. The role that God calls the family to perform in history derives from what the family is; its role represents the dynamic and existential development of what it is. Each family finds within itself a summons that cannot be ignored, and that specifies both its dignity and its responsibility: family, become what you are.

Accordingly, the family must go back to the "beginning" of God's creative act, if it is to attain self-knowledge and self-realization in accordance with the inner truth not only of what it is but also of what it does in history. And since in God's plan it has been established as an "intimate community of life and love," the family has the mission to become more and more what it is, that is to say, a community of life and love, in an effort that will find fulfillment, as will everything created and redeemed, in the Kingdom of God. Looking at it in such a way as to reach its very roots, we must say that the essence and role of the family are in the final analysis specified by love. Hence the family has the mission to guard, reveal and communicate love, and this is a living reflection of and a real sharing in God's love for humanity and the love of Christ the Lord for the Church His bride.

Every particular task of the family is an expressive and concrete actuation of that fundamental mission. We must therefore go deeper into the unique riches of the family's mission and probe its contents, which are both manifold and unified.

Thus, with love as its point of departure and making constant reference to it, the recent Synod emphasized four general tasks for the family:

1. Forming a community of persons
2. Serving life
3. Participating in the development of society
4. Sharing in the life and mission of the Church

I encourage you to consider reading *Familiaris Consortio* in its entirety and pray for the graces to be able to live toward the goal John Paul II outlines for each of us. You can find it online at the Vatican website.

Praying Your Pregnancy

Guide me in my marriage, Lord, and help me to keep you at the center, even as our family grows larger, distractions increase, and challenges appear. Hold me close to what you have in mind for our family. Lead me to a greater fulfillment of my roles of wife and mother. Amen.

CHAPTER 8

Week 12 (Fetal Age: 10 Weeks)

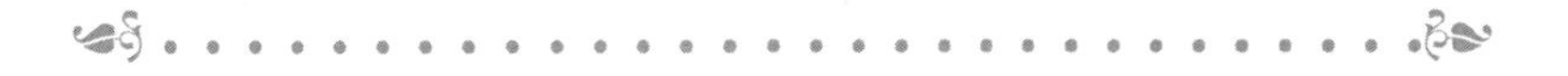

Depression during Pregnancy

Did you know that depression during pregnancy could be the most common medical complication found in pregnant women, according to some experts? Before I read about it, I had no idea.

The silence I experienced about depression during pregnancy isn't uncommon. After all, isn't it good that you're pregnant? Aren't you supposed to be glowing and happy and floating on air?

If you're facing depression, don't be afraid to ask for help. Talk to your doctor, midwife, or other medical professional. Ask your husband if he's noticed any differences, anything that alarms him.

It's not easy to ask for help, but if you are facing depression, you need to ask for help, and you need to take it a step further: you need to accept help. Sometimes, having someone to talk to—a trusted friend, a spiritual director, a family member—can help. Sometimes reaching out to others can take you beyond yourself.

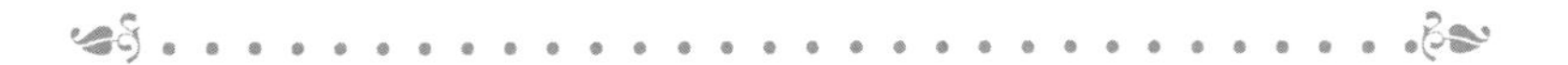

THOUGH STILL TINY, YOUR BABY HAS NEARLY doubled in size in the last three weeks![13] She's now moving around all the time and can squint, open her mouth, and move her fingers and toes.[14]

Are you starting to feel a little better? In many cases, entering the second trimester means that any of the ickiness you were experiencing has improved. This may be the point that you start to feel a little bit of the pregnancy glow. If not, you can take comfort knowing that you've made it a third of the way: you're getting there! It takes longer for some women to feel better.

TIPS FOR HANDLING DEPRESSION DURING PREGNANCY:

- Shower and get dressed every day, even if you don't have to.
- Eat regular meals, even if you're not hungry.
- Keep a day-night schedule, where you're awake in the day and asleep at night.
- Exercise, even if it's nothing more than opening the blinds and walking around the block slowly.
- Make meaningful social contact every single day, whether through a phone call or e-mail or a visit to a friend.

At some point soon, your medical provider will probably ask you about testing. Do you want to know if your child might have Down syndrome? My doctor always asks me if it will make any difference, and I always reply, "Nope. We'll take what God has given us." At that point, they don't push me to have the testing. (Some doctors will still push. Be prepared to stand by your decision.)

My bravado, though, is just that. I have a great fear, when I'm pregnant, of things being wrong with my baby. What's wrong with my outlook, though, is the perspective that so many of the things being tested are "wrong." Down syndrome is far from the worst thing that a child could deal with during life.

Whether you opt for the testing or decide to pass on it, remember that the baby within you is a person created in God's image, just as we all are. God has given you this baby.

It's usually at about this point in a pregnancy that things become really real for me. For one thing, my usual clothes aren't fitting quite right, and I have no patience for squeezing into jeans when they won't button. For another, I never fail to get a sinus infection or a cold at about this point in pregnancy. Because so much of what helps me is on the no-no list for pregnant women, I'm aware of that new life in a whole new way.

Hearing the heartbeat, too, makes the reality of another person inside me real. I begin to wonder about my baby's future: Will she have her father's eyes, her sibling's forehead, or her grandfather's charisma?

With those questions come others, many of them rooted in anxiety. Will my baby make it? Will we have an unpleasant surprise? Will we be able to make it through whatever's ahead of us?

If you find yourself with a seed of anxiety growing in you, try spending the week in Mary's presence. Think of her as a person to whom you can go and simply spend time—just as my children migrate to whatever room I'm working in, and I tend to visit my mother-in-law when I need to feel better. Feel safe and comforted just knowing she's there for you. While you pray this week's decade of the Rosary, ask her to calm you and to hold you close to her son. Trust that he will carry you when you need it and that you need never wonder about the future.

Walking with Mary: The Proclamation of the Kingdom

The idea of God's kingdom seems so distant from the daily chaos that keeps me juggling. I end my days out of breath and wonder how I can create more hours in a day.

Father Benedict Groeschel, in his audio reflections, *The Rosary Is a Place*, describes the kingdom coming in our hearts as the only place it can truly come. This meditation on the kingdom of heaven reminds me that conversion doesn't happen "out there." What's important is what's in me. That's all I can control, all I can offer, and all I can do.

Jesus offers us the kingdom of heaven, but that's no good if we don't long for it, if we can't picture a place that's better than what we have here on earth. Do we really desire God's will? Does his plan for our life correspond with how we are living, with what we are doing, and with where we are going?

God's kingdom comes to me by way of the small people in my life, those who often make demands of me all day long. They are often ungrateful, and they don't usually show me much—if any—recognition. They are, in fact, much the way I am toward my heavenly Father.

Just as they assume I will take care of their needs, I often forget to turn to the Lord with more than a demand for help. How often do I make time for the kingdom to be formed in my heart and manifested in my life? When do I sit still long enough for the still, small voice to be heard above the activity around me? What can I do to make room for the kingdom to come in my own heart?

One Small Step

The proclamation of the kingdom reminds us that sin distances us from the kingdom of heaven. Sin is a choice we make, a step we take away from God.

Until I became Catholic, I didn't really know what forgiveness meant. Since then, the sacrament of Reconciliation has been the sacrament I love to hate and hate to love. It's hard to go to confession, I know! But once I'm there and after I leave, I'm so relieved.

What happened to that sin that drove me there? It's washed away, and in my penance I find the opportunity to unite myself more closely with Christ, who bore my sin on the cross (CCC, 1460). I am repaired, healed, restored; I place myself before God and his mercy (CCC, 1469–70) and come out of it a better person, resolved to try again to be the person God intends me to be.

Just as sin has a damaging effect, reaching far beyond the sinner who commits the sin, so too Reconciliation has a healing effect on the entire Church. The Catechism says that it "has also a revitalizing effect on the life of the Church which suffered from the sin of one of her members. Re-established or strengthened in the communion of saints, the sinner is made stronger by the exchange of spiritual goods among all the living members of the Body of Christ" (*CCC*, 1469).

In other words, it's not just about me. Pregnancy is a master's degree in giving of your very self for someone else, and it can lead us to better appreciate the gifts of the sacrament of Reconciliation.

Right now, nothing is between you and your baby. This is the only time you will have this intimacy with your little one, and someday, she may run far away from you. Imagine reaching after her as she runs away from you, pursuing her own interests and getting herself hurt and bruised in the process. Wouldn't you do anything to take away the pain, the sorrow, and the hurt?

God pursues you in the same way. You are his beloved child, and you exist for him as though you are the only person in the world. In a world where we're told that "nothing is personal," here's something that's so personal that it's made just for you.

God made you, and he longs to hold you close. Accept his hand this week and take advantage of the gift of the sacraments he's left for you. Don't waste a minute; do it now, before you can talk yourself out of it.

Faith Focus

There are days when I'm so distracted that even a guided prayer like the Rosary isn't possible. It's then that I'm so grateful for the scriptural Rosary. In this method of praying the Rosary, there are verses from the Bible inserted between each Hail Mary. Not only does it keep my focus on the mystery

I'm praying, it also teaches me about the biblical roots of each mystery.

There are many versions of this available, whether as an app for your smartphone or device, on websites, as audio downloads, or even in book format. My appreciation and focus for each of the mysteries of the Rosary have grown because of the use of a scripture verse or passage before each Hail Mary. I find myself memorizing scripture, and though it feels accidental, when I find some of those verses seeming to just pop into my head throughout a rough day, I know who's speaking, and I feel the comfort of his voice.

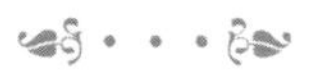

Praying Your Pregnancy

Hi there, God. It's me again. Seems I'm struggling a lot these days, and I guess I need to tell you more about it. Growing another person isn't easy, but, for that matter, life isn't easy. Give me the grace to come to you this week and accept your embrace. Amen.

CHAPTER 9

Week 13 (Fetal Age: 11 Weeks)

YOU'RE AT THE POINT IN YOUR PREGNANCY WHERE your uterus is going to be growing more noticeably. It can't be avoided, really, since your baby needs more room. He's the size of a peach this week, and his head is a huge portion of his body mass right now. Right now, his head is almost half of the crown-to-rump length, but the rest of him will be catching up in the coming weeks. These developments have made his face look more human, with eyes and ears nearly in their correct positions.

If you haven't started wearing maternity clothes or a bellyband yet, you probably will soon. Your waist will be inching outward more and more as your body stretches to accommodate your growing baby. As this happens, you might struggle with the idea of losing your figure. If so, try considering that the stretch marks and changes in your body as a sign of God's love. Within each crease and difference in your body is proof of sacrifice—the sacrifice you are making to grow your baby and will continue to make, as he grows older. Your post-baby body can be a beacon of hope to you, because you provide a witness to love by carrying a child within you. You have earned your new body, and you should see it as beautiful for what it is: a nurturing, safe place for your child.

Walking with Mary: The Institution of the Eucharist

I often wonder what Mary truly looked like as a whole person. I don't think our statues and paintings do her justice, in part because we don't see her as an entire person, but are limited by the visual. There's no interaction with a cold, still statue. You don't see the twinkle in her eye, experience the subtlety of her stance, or hear the tone of her voice.

I've known many women who probably wouldn't grace the cover of *Vogue*, yet they are no less beautiful to me. Their beauty comes from within and reaches past their wrinkles and bodily imperfections to the way they embrace their role in life and encourage others around them. In these women, I see that each gray hair is a stepping-stone to sainthood and each stretch mark the ultimate sign of love.

Unfortunately, this isn't the message sent by our culture. Instead, we are told that truly beautiful models aren't good enough; they are airbrushed to flawlessness before they grace the pages of the magazines we see in the checkout lines we stand in every day. These images of so-called perfection set us up for failure by making us desire something that doesn't exist. The result is a desire to avoid anything that can cause imperfections as defined by our culture. But our definitions are skewed. We need a lesson in understanding how giving is what makes us beautiful, and when we cooperate with God to give life to another, we become the truest depiction of beauty.

Mary shows us the beauty of giving and sacrifice. She gave up her body in pregnancy. She carried Jesus within herself, and she took him to her cousin Elizabeth when she went to serve and give. She carried him in her heart as he walked the streets of Jerusalem, burdened with the weight of the Cross. She carried him to everyone around her after he ascended to heaven.

We carry Jesus, too. At every Mass, we receive the Eucharist, which is Jesus. It's hard for me to think of that small round host as Jesus. Getting too literal with it makes me feel a little sick, in truth, for the same reason that many of his disciples left him after he said, "Whoever eats my flesh and drinks my blood remains in me and I in him" (Jn 6:56).

But I can't let my aversions keep me from the gift Jesus offers me. The Eucharist is my fuel for the hard work ahead of me, whether it's the mothering of a child in utero or the mothering of a child in front of me. The many sacrifices we are called to make in any given day are best handled when we are basking in the graces of Jesus himself. Jesus gave up his body, just as you are giving up yours to carry this child. You will give up so much in the months ahead to bring life into the world, and then you will give in many other ways to nurture that life. The physical changes you experience last at least two lifetimes—yours and your baby's.

Just as the baby within you changes you, stretching your body to grow and your life to expand, so Jesus will change you when he is within you. Some change requires our cooperation—the baby within you is healthier when you take care of yourself, and so Jesus can work through you better with your help—but you will be changed, regardless.

The Eucharist is the source and summit of our life as Christians (*CCC*, 1324). It's our strength and our energy. It's also a reminder to us of the work we're to do with love, of how we're to live the life of sacrifice and carry Jesus to those around us, as Mary did. How can we truly be more like Jesus, more like Mary, and more like the people God intends for us to be?

One Small Step

The sacrament of Holy Orders brings us our priests and deacons. Your parish probably has at least one man who's been ordained as a priest or deacon, and you might have more than one.

I didn't fully appreciate what these men did for our church communities until I worked in our parish office. Though we have a small rural parish, our priest doesn't hesitate to get involved with teaching at a nearby high school, offering confessions whenever he's asked, showing up at our religious-education classes, and conducting a series of Bible studies that never fail to be insightful and inspiring.

Our deacon, who has a family of his own, has been involved in many ministries throughout our diocese, and every single week he can be found at a soup kitchen in the metropolitan area. He makes frequent bread runs to a large chain store near us and is also a hospital chaplain.

Both of these men are involved in ways that are invisible to many people in the parish. I don't know the full extent of their ministry, and I suspect they wouldn't want me to know. For them—and for most ordained men—it's not important to get the credit. They don't do it for the glory. They do it for God.

They "give up" for each of us, the Body of Christ in the Church, just as Jesus gave up his life, just as you are giving up your body throughout pregnancy and beyond. When you find yourself struggling with the changes to your appearance and your body, which you may perceive as "ugly," think of the inner beauty that causes each of us to glow with the light of Christ. We carry this light through our obedience to our vocational calls, whether or not those around us are able to see and appreciate it for what it is or not.

This week, why not invite your priest or deacon (and his wife, if he has one) to dinner or write them a thank-you card? Express how they inspire you as you stand on the threshold of new life, and give them the gift of your ongoing prayer and support.

Faith Focus

> So when he had washed their feet (and) put his garments back on and reclined at table again, he said to them, "Do you realize what I have done for you? You call me 'teacher' and 'master,' and rightly so, for indeed I am. If I, therefore, the master and teacher, have washed your feet, you ought to wash one another's feet. I have given you a model to follow, so that as I have done for you, you should also do." (Jn 13:10–15)

On the night he gave his body and blood for us in the Eucharist, he also performed the washing of his apostles' feet, reminding us that there is always work to be done. Open your arms for the work in front of you, and ask God for the grace to cooperate with his plan for your life. Allow Christ to be your guide as you embrace the physical changes occurring, and give up your very self throughout pregnancy and motherhood.

Praying Your Pregnancy

God, help me to stop and see you in the midst of the many changes taking place around me. Draw me closer to you, and let me feel your peace within me, especially after I receive you in the Eucharist. Guide me toward a joyful acceptance of who I am, how I am, and the way I look, now and in the future. Amen.

CHAPTER 10

Week 14 (Fetal Age: 12 Weeks)

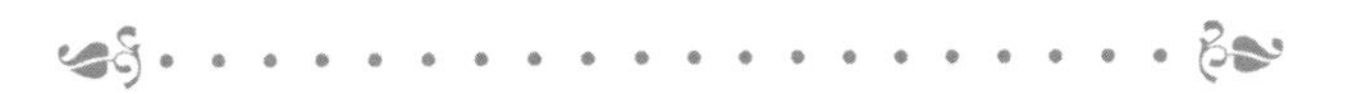

ARE YOU STARTING TO FEEL LIKE YOU'RE ON A LONG journey? Do you have a sneaking feeling of guilt that you're not enjoying and loving every moment of pregnancy?

I know many women who have struggled with infertility and loss of children, women who long to hold a baby. It's those women who come to mind when I find myself less than halfway through a pregnancy and hating it.

I don't hate the baby, mind you, or even the pregnancy itself. I hate the discomfort, the pain, the hurdles of exhaustion and sickness. I hate that my favorite foods make me vomit and that complaining makes me selfish. I hate the resentment that creeps in and the mess that grows in my house.

Pregnancy is not easy for many of us. It is often not fun. In fact, for me, it's been a bit of foreshadowing for how parenthood is.

But you know what? Even if it seems hard and not enjoyable now, it is so worth it. That growing baby bump you're hauling around in front of you has already changed your life and will only continue to do so. Being a parent is hard work, but it's also the most important work you'll ever be blessed to undertake. You might hate the specifics (I do many days), but you are growing the kingdom of God in the most important way possible: through your domestic church and by cooperating with the graces of your vocation.

There's a lot going on in your body right now, and your hormones create a brew that is sometimes unpleasant. Don't lose sight, though, of the role you play. Don't forget the importance of this cross and the love that's coming down from heaven for you. Ask for the grace to carry your cross. Beg for help from above. Then keep watch and step back, because you're sure to be amazed at the result of your trust.

Walking with Mary: The Agony in the Garden

When I read about the apostles falling asleep in the garden, I always shake my head, because I can relate. I've fallen asleep in the most unlikely places, including crowded sports stadiums and movie theaters.

When I'm asleep, I can escape from my dread and fear of the future. At least, that's the theory. When my dreams turn on me, then I know it's time for something more drastic, something like turning to God.

Jesus did ask for the cup of suffering to pass him by. He didn't want to suffer. Neither do I! What's important here, though, is that he finished the thought with, "Thy will be done." In my parlance, that equals, "Please, please, please, make it easier! Make it not hurt! But if it has to be bad, then carry me on your back."

There's only one place to turn with my dread, and that's heavenward. There's only one source of true comfort that will give me actual peace, and that's God. Facing the long journey of pregnancy and the ultimate end of labor overwhelms me every single time. I can't sleep through it, though I'll try at first. I can't avoid it; I must walk through it.

Jesus doesn't condemn the apostles for sleeping in the garden, but he doesn't let them off the hook either. How much better prepared would they have been if they had been awake and praying? How can I learn from them? How can I turn to Jesus in my suffering?

One Small Step

One year, one of my favorite bloggers mentioned that she was doing a one-word resolution for the year. I love resolutions any time of the year, and I embraced the word "peace" for that year. A friend bought me a small sign and a steppingstone with "peace" emblazoned on them, and I put them where I would see them every day.

Now when I see them, years later, I remember how focusing on that one word helped me so much. It was a tumultuous year, but somehow, I felt close to God and that he was very much in control.

In my faith life, I continue to find a great wellspring of faith from sitting with Jesus during eucharistic adoration. Though our parish has a program with exposition (where the host is displayed in a special, very fancy, holder called a monstrance), I sometimes just stop by the church and sit in front of the tabernacle. Jesus is really present. He holds me close and offers me the very best kind of peace.

Go sit with Jesus this week. Though he is with you wherever you are, make a special visit and spend a while with him. If you can only spare fifteen minutes, he'll take it. If you have an hour, spend that. If it's a sacrifice for you, consider that you're making an investment in the most important relationship in your life.

Faith Focus

She would wake, screaming, and I would lie in bed unable to go back to sleep as I listened to my husband hold her. Some nights, I was the one who got up and soothed her.

My daughter has never been a good sleeper. She was three before she slept through the night regularly, and it took me years to accept that it wasn't my fault, that nothing my in my mothering skill set could change how she was. When she began to wake screaming, though, something had to change.

It started on a whim, because I was desperate: one night, my daughter and I began praying the Saint Michael prayer before bed. She memorized it sooner than I did, but both of us turn to that prayer now whenever we are scared.

> Saint Michael the Archangel, defend us in battle,
> Be our protection against the malice and snares of the devil.
> May God rebuke him, we humbly pray.
> And do thou, oh Prince of the heavenly host, by the divine power,
> Thrust into hell Satan and all evil spirits
> who prowl about the world, seeking the ruin of souls.

At the end of the prayer, before saying "Amen," we often add a specific intention, such as "Stay close to me and keep me from being afraid," or "Help me be safe and have good dreams." Consider praying and asking Saint Michael to defend you from the nagging fears and persistent concerns that face you during pregnancy.

• • •

Praying Your Pregnancy

Dear Jesus, I want peace. I want to avoid the cup of suffering. I want to walk with you, but the way is rocky and hard. Show me the simple way to your arms, and keep me close while I grow this new person within me. Give me the grace to do your will every day. Amen.

CHAPTER 11

Week 15
(Fetal Age: 13 Weeks)

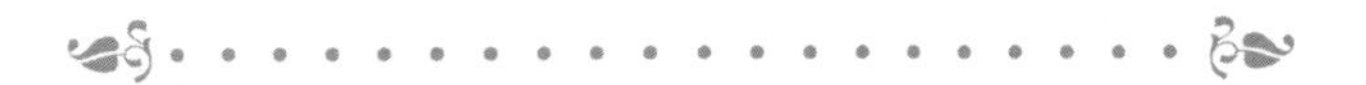

Boy, Girl, or Surprise?

I was shocked, with my first pregnancy, when my husband was the one who insisted on finding out the gender. With our second pregnancy, it was the same. And guess what? With our third pregnancy, the one where I felt most strongly that it might be fun to wait and see, he just couldn't help it.

"I have to know!" he told me. "It drives me crazy that the doctor knows and I don't!"

For him, it's a matter of excitement. I've found, for myself and especially as a non-baby person, that knowing the baby's gender helps me to begin to think of the baby as a little person. Though they were in me and thus already real, something about knowing the proper pronoun helped me connect with my new role as the mother.

On the other hand, I have a good friend who has never found out the gender of her babies, and I don't think she will in any future pregnancies, either. She insists that it's her greatest reward after labor. Not only does she get a prize—the baby—but she also gets to find out the answer to the gender mystery!

Whatever you decide, I encourage you to smile about it. There will be no shortage of people to subtly criticize you or hint that you are making a mistake. Don't let that get you down: stick to your decision, and enjoy its benefits.

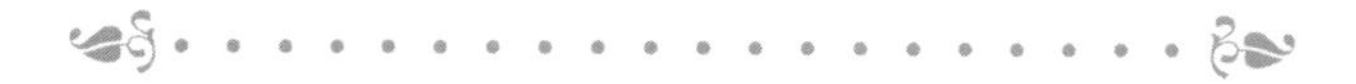

IT'S HARD TO BELIEVE THAT YOUR BABY, WHO STARTED as a clump of cells, is now the size of a softball. There's a fine hair covering her body, and her skin's so thin that the blood vessels show through. Her bones have formed and are hardening as they retain calcium.

My favorite part about this point in the pregnancy is that the baby may be sucking her thumb. Though I know that the baby is a human from the point of conception, it's when she starts sucking her thumb that I start to picture an actual baby instead of just a formless mass. I was a thumb-sucker until an embarrassingly late age, and this baby and I have something tangible in common.

Even if the world can't tell for sure that you're pregnant, you definitely know by the differences in your body, especially your lower abdominal area. Can you feel your uterus below your belly button?

Walking with Mary: Scourging at the Pillar

When I worked in our parish office, I brought my first baby with me, just as she was learning to crawl. One day I got insight into the scourging at the pillar. I was talking to an older mom on the phone, and she said, "Every time I talk badly about someone, it's a cut in Jesus's back."

Her words gave make whole new perspective on the scourging and my own actions. How many times do I hurt others without knowing it, without really thinking about the effects of my actions or words, and without even considering them at all?

That older mom also made me think about Jesus's back. I don't really know what a scourging involves, but I've seen the movie *The Passion of the Christ* and I've read about it. It's enough to turn my stomach and to make me want to think about something else, almost anything else.

Jesus did not, however, fight back. He didn't accuse his torturers or cast an evil eye at them. He accepted what they were doing. He loved them in spite of it. He forgave them before they were finished.

Where was Mary during the scourging? Did she watch it? Was she overcome with bitterness and hatred toward her son's torturers?

When I think of the Mother of God watching her son being beaten to a bloody pulp, I can't help but wonder if it's a human trait to want to lash back, to fight, and to get even. But that's not what Jesus did, and I suspect it's not what his mother did either.

When I'm pregnant, I often find myself drudging through old hurts and painful memories. I embroil myself in all the ways I've been wronged and can all too easily find myself an emotional mess. Looking to Jesus at the pillar, then, gives me a focus and a path to forgiveness.

One Small Step

Sacramentals are "sacred signs instituted by the Church" that "prepare men to receive the fruit of the sacraments and sanctify different circumstances of life" (*CCC*, 1677). They include items such as rosaries, holy water, crucifixes, icons, and articles that remind us of our faith.

Whether it's the picture that hangs in our kitchen or the medal in our pocket, the crucifix around our neck or the holy water in our car, sacramentals can make our faith come to life by reminding us of it during the odd moments of our day. My priest once shared that he keeps a flat crucifix on his desk so that, in the middle of the day when he's trying to straighten things and going through papers, he has the reminder to stop and pray.

This week use a sacramental in a new way—a holy card in the book you're reading, a rosary under your pillow, a crucifix on your wall—and use it to turn to God. Embrace the call to holiness within your vocation, and grow closer to the path God has called you to follow.

Faith Focus

Within each Catholic church is some version of Stations of the Cross. They're sacramentals in the church building and a prayer tradition that has a lot to teach us. This devotion started in the fourth century and is made up of fourteen scenes from the passion of Christ. Each scene is intended to help us make a pilgrimage to the sites of Jesus's suffering and death, even if we can't travel to the Holy Land physically.

During Lent, my parish has a tradition of praying the Stations every Friday night. I've only attended once or twice, but each time I've been immensely moved. I've prayed the Stations many times on my own, though, and have even used time at adoration to walk around the church and pray them while looking up at the paintings hanging on our church walls.

There's horror in going deeply into Jesus's suffering and agony, but there's also comfort. Pregnancy isn't easy, and praying the Stations of the Cross helps me get beyond the temptation to think that a man couldn't possibly understand, even if he is God.

Praying Your Pregnancy

Jesus, I'm excited to be a mother, and yet I'm scared. I'm full of hope, and yet I'm also full of the pain from my past. Heal me, hold me, and lead me to you. Use my pregnancy as a way to help me grow closer to you. Amen.

CHAPTER 12

Week 16 (Fetal Age: 14 Weeks)

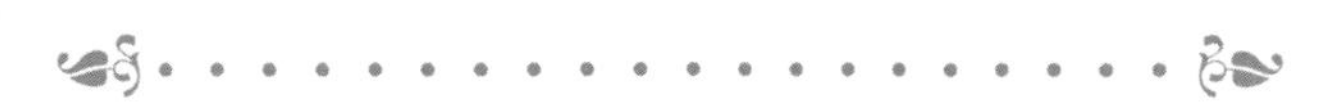

The Unexpected Child

By Leticia Velasquez

I had already had two births and three miscarriages when I was expecting my sixth baby at age thirty-nine. Midway through this pregnancy, while I was at Mass, I had a spiritual insight that my baby had Down syndrome. I was stunned and incredulous. I felt completely inadequate and unable to raise a child with special needs. Only living saints were given such children, I thought. I would never be equal to the demands of raising such a child, I was sure of it. Besides, I feared that my marriage would collapse if our child were especially needy. God would never choose us to raise a special-needs child. Of that I was certain.

"I want you to accept this child as a gift from my hand when you receive me" were the words I heard in my heart in response to my panic that my child had Down syndrome. I was in line for Holy Communion, and my "yes, Lord" was accompanied by a flood of tears and a condition, "please bring my husband along for the ride." Hardly the unconditional "let it be done to me according to Your will" of Our Blessed Mother!

Four months later, Christina surprised her doctors when she was born with Down syndrome. Even though our Lord had prepared me, I still wallowed in a bit of self-pity; then I picked up my tiny baby and became her mother. I became a different mother than I was for my other daughters, a special mother. God was faithful in giving the graces my husband and I needed to parent our special baby just as we needed them. I look back with gratitude on the first days of her life. Our Lord was surely carrying us in his arms.

Ten years later, Christina is a happy third grader and the apple of her daddy's eye. She has health issues and developmental challenges, but they are not what you notice when she beams at you and wraps you in her bear hug. You see a beautiful, loving little girl, who is a living sign of Jesus's love for my family. Not only that, she is a sign of hope for the world, that God doesn't love us for what we are, but who we are: his beloved children.

That's what Jesus may be trying to show you through your tears. That he holds your child's future in his hand, not the doctor's. They can tell you symptoms and statistics they learned in medical school; they can't tell you about that joy that we have come to know in our special-needs child. Your child is a gift from God's hand, and only good comes from our Father. This child may be your elevator to heaven.

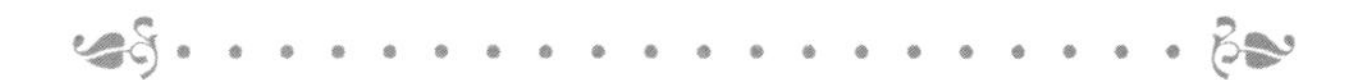

HE HAS FINGERNAILS AND THEY LOOK LIKE fingernails. He has a hairline, too, and perhaps the start of a kicking regime as he moves his arms and legs more frequently. Maybe you feel the little fluttering movement of your baby within you, but maybe not quite yet.

When I first felt a baby move within me, with my first pregnancy, it was a quiet morning at adoration, just Jesus and me. The baby was probably moving and kicking quite a bit for me to notice the tiny stirrings, and I was amazed.

Though I'm not naturally a baby person—even, sometimes, with my own babies—even I can't deny the wonder of another human being moving around inside my body. Later in the pregnancy, such movement loses its appeal and might even become painful.

You may be experiencing headaches and congestion in place of (or even in addition to) your nausea, and you might also shake your head when people tell you that there's a glow to you. It's difficult to smile and remain gracious when you're not feeling well. Focusing too much on the physical discomfort can keep you from considering the miracle within you.

It's hard, for me at least, to just say, "Thanks" when people tell me I look great when I'm pregnant. One of the reasons might be that my natural worry is fed by the comments about how I look. One person thinks I look tiny, while another asks if I'm having twins or due in five minutes.

It's made me realize the great humility I can learn during the journey through pregnancy: letting go and trusting God has rarely had a more literal application in my life. I have to look hard, sometimes, to find the inner radiance that others seem to see so clearly and easily, but even the seeking keeps me focusing on the positive. I don't have to deny the hard parts of pregnancy, but when I immerse myself in them, I lose sight of the remarkable person within me.

Walking with Mary: Crowning with Thorns

There's a saying that I remember using on the grade-school playground: "Sticks and stones can break my bones, but words can never hurt me." We usually stuck our tongues out at the end and took off running.

I've found, though, that words can and do hurt, and they stick like thorns in my mind, twisting and turning. They're hard to forget, harder still to forgive. They linger when the event that hosted them is long forgotten.

Jesus faced mockery and sarcasm from the soldiers as they forced a crown of thorns on his head. I've felt the barbs of others' well-intended words and ill-advised comments circle my head and drive deep into my consciousness by my own obsession with recalling them.

Jesus' response is to love them. He forgives them so completely, it's as though the offense never happened.

Could Jesus have learned this example of gentleness from his earthly parents? I have noticed, in my own children, the way they will imitate so much of what I do, encompassing both my best and worst habits in their own actions.

From Jesus, I see a mirror of how Mary must have treated other people. In his love, I glimpse her love. In his forgiveness in the face of pain and hatred, I see her embodiment of the gospel as she raised him.

When do I turn into one of the soldiers, using my tongue to crown someone with mockery or sarcasm, criticism or gossip, recrimination or contempt? How often do I forgive . . . and how often do I ask for forgiveness? What could I do to wear my own crown for the glory of God and the example of humility?

One Small Step

I made a resolution, many years ago, to do my best not to talk badly about my husband. Ever.

Most of the time, it's pretty easy. There are times, though, that I catch myself longing to criticize something about him, and I have to remember this resolution. There are other times that I fail.

This week, recommit to your marriage by resolving to say only positive things about your spouse.

Faith Focus

One of the best ways for me to learn about my new Catholic faith was to begin working in my parish office. I had been Catholic for a few years at that point, but was newly married and full of excitement about my novel faith. Every day, I had a chance to ask Father all the questions I could think of and to glean answers to questions I never even thought to ask. I also learned some of the inner workings and gained a comfort level with the Church that I appreciate now.

The topic of Mass intentions was one I never understood—and never thought of—until I worked in the parish office. Simply put, each Mass can be offered for a specific intention. In many parishes, you schedule this through the parish office and offer a stipend in exchange. Years ago (and in some countries, this is still true), the stipends were part of the priest's salary, and a much-needed part! Now, most priests are paid a salary, and stipends are additional income.

In addition, I learned that you can offer your Mass yourself. So when I go to Mass, I can offer it for the repose of my aunt or even for my husband's struggles at work. It can be my own private offering, or it can be done formally through the parish office.

Having a Mass offered is like a prayer on steroids. Everyone at that Mass is praying for that intention along with you. You don't need to be present at the Mass you've scheduled through the office. If you're offering a Mass you attend, it's more of a private commitment.

Masses can also be offered for living people, and I've learned over the years to put these down as a "special intention" without specific names, lest people come and, with their well-meaning questions, raise alarm or worry (especially if the person in question doesn't know you're having the Mass offered for him or her). You can also offer Masses for an intention, such as for your marriage or in thanksgiving for an answered prayer.

Mass brings us together as the Body of Christ, and when you offer your Mass—either formally through the parish office or personally, just in your own offering—you unite your prayer with the rest of the family. I've found that it's made great changes in me, and that, with those changes, I can sometimes even find the grace to accept God's answer when it's different from what I expect or think I want.

Praying Your Pregnancy

Sometimes I forget the power of words in the flurry of movement around me, Lord. Help me this week to be still and treasure the small person inside me, whether or not I feel any movement. Guide me closer to you, so that I may give glory to you every moment of my day. Amen.

CHAPTER 13

Week 17 (Fetal Age: 15 Weeks)

JUST A FEW SHORT MONTHS AGO, YOUR BABY COULD hardly be seen with the naked eye. This week, she's about the size of your hand spread open wide. She's also starting to form fat, which will help her heat production and metabolism.

This is the point when you become conscious of your baby's presence, because you're probably feeling her movement more frequently. Though you may not feel these movements every day, they are happening more, probably in the quiet times of your day or night.

At this point, you may also be experiencing leg cramps. I remember waking in the middle of the night with some of the most intense charley horses I've ever had. Eating bananas might help, and you might want to just make a habit of chugging water. I've read too that calcium intake can help.

It wasn't until I had some strange pains during my third pregnancy that I started to get a glimpse of why people were always telling me to take it easy and rest during pregnancy. With my first two, I didn't really change anything in my life. I just kept going. When I started to have sharp, stabbing pains in my side at about this point in that third pregnancy, though, I gave in to a bit of worry and called my mother-in-law and my best friend.

Both of them advised me to rest, something I never do well. The pains went away, but with that pregnancy, they would come back periodically when I overextended myself (which was more often than I'd like to admit). I didn't ever find myself on bed rest, but I had a glimpse of how complicated things could get very quickly.

It's not easy to slow down and rest. For some of us, sitting still is akin to torture, especially when there are other people to care for and lots of work to do. I always think I can just keep going. It's hard to slow down when you know how much time is in front of you with this pregnancy.

There's a gift in the slowing down, though. Try it, and see. Cuddle up with your toddler or your husband, and take a nap. Grab a Rosary, and let the dishes wait while you spend a few moments with a mom who understands your journey. Stepping back now will give you the endurance you'll need for what's to come.

Walking with Mary: Carrying the Cross

She leaned into her husband in the front row, their two young girls sprawled between them. The older daughter, who was around five, had an idea of what was going on, but the younger daughter was only three. She just saw a lot of crying and a baby in a casket.

My husband's family buried a baby before we were married, and the image stayed with me throughout my own pregnancies. Whenever I felt like things were too hard for me during pregnancy, I thought of the baby my sister-in-law held only briefly and whom Mama Mary continues to cuddle in heaven. Whenever I was tempted to complain about pregnancy or reflect on what a pain the baby would be for the first year of life, I thought of the women I knew who struggle valiantly and courageously with infertility.

Our crosses are uniquely our own. You would probably laugh if I told you the things that make my days almost harder than I can bear, and I might smile to hear about your difficulties. Then again, we might cause each other to sob out of compassion.

So many of the crosses I have are made heavier by my approach to them. Instead of just walking along and dealing with them, I spend energy complaining, dreading, and trying to avoid them. Rather than offer them to God or—better yet—rather than asking him to help me, I try to do it just like my toddler insists, "By myself!"

When Jesus carried his cross, it wasn't easy. But it did end. Our crosses aren't forever. If there's an aspect of your pregnancy that is a cross for you, turn to this mystery in a special way. Ask Mary to help you turn your focus toward the One who stands ready to help you carry it.

One Small Step

We're told to "refrain from engaging in work or activities that hinder the worship owed to God, the joy proper to the Lord's Day, the performance of the works of mercy, and the appropriate relaxation of mind and body" on Sundays and the other holy days of obligation (*CCC*, 2185). It's easier said than done these days, until it becomes a habit.

In my own life, I've found that Sunday rest equals a decrease (or a complete lack) of screen time, especially my computer screen. The work I do that's not family related, which I mostly do from home, usually involves my laptop. And so, on Sundays, I try to keep that laptop closed. Though I sometimes sneak time on my tablet or even sit down with my family to enjoy a movie, I am using the screens for something other than work.

Another thing I try to avoid on Sundays is shopping. Why make someone else have to work on Sunday? There are times it is unavoidable (usually because of my own lack of planning), but many times, the shopping I would do on Sunday can be done on Saturday or through the week.

God rested on the seventh day after spending six days creating the world. He's our model. Though our Sabbath is now on the first day of the week in honor of the Resurrection, we still need a day of rest. It's good for us psychologically, it's good for our families, and it's good for our souls.

So, this week, clear your calendar on Sunday. Spend the day lounging, if that's what recharges you. Remember to pray, too, and to look heavenward in thanksgiving for a day to recuperate from the work of the week. Mass should be a part of your observation, whether you go to the Saturday vigil or sometime on Sunday.

That said, you might still find yourself doing household chores or laundry. Try, though, to arrange things so that you can truly rest from whatever it is you call work.

Faith Focus

> Then the Lord said: "Go out and stand on the mountain before the Lord; the Lord will be passing by." A strong and heavy wind was rending the mountains and crushing rocks before the Lord—but the Lord was not in the wind. After the wind, there was an earthquake—but the Lord was not in the earthquake. After the earthquake, there was fire—but the Lord was not in the fire. After the fire, there was a tiny whispering sound. When he heard this, Elijah hid his face in his cloak and went and stood at the entrance of the cave. (1 Kgs 19:11–13)

Elijah was yearning to speak to God, and God agreed to meet with him. You'd expect fanfare and some sort of noise, wouldn't you? And yet, in this passage we read that the Lord was a "tiny whispering sound."

How often do you sit in silence? Do you ever turn off everything—all the screens, all the background noises, and all the electronic distractions—and sit in God's presence? You can do it at your kitchen table, in your parish church, or in the car as you wait at a soccer game or during lunch.

Silence is important. We need to hear God's voice, but he does not shout. He won't push his way in past our crowded and distracted attention. When we carve out time for God in silence, we'll see the fruit of it spread throughout our lives. It impacts everyone.

It's not easy, and it may just be a few minutes at first. Grow an appetite for silent time with God. Approach it with no agenda and no expectation. Open yourself to hearing the light silent sound of the Holy Spirit in your life.

Praying Your Pregnancy

God, there is so much noise and busyness in my life. There is always something more to do, always something waiting for my attention, always more, more, more! Help me to stop and see you in the midst of chaos. Draw me closer to you and show me your tender love. Give me the courage to sit in silence with you, and help me to turn my crosses to you. Amen.

CHAPTER 14

Week 18 (Fetal Age: 16 Weeks)

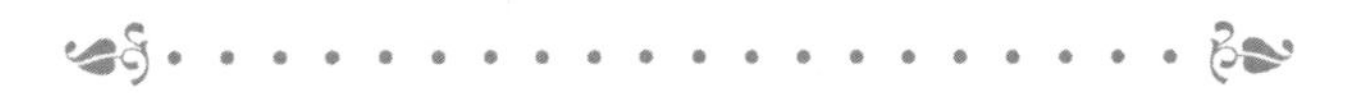

Keeping Daddy Involved

Daddy is half the reason the baby exists, and yet it sometimes takes extra effort to keep him involved during the pregnancy. For one thing, it's not his body that has a baby inside it.

I'm not any better at keeping my husband involved with my pregnancies than anyone else is. In fact, I can think of plenty of ways I could improve if we have a next time around.

Thanks to the Internet and the many cool apps available for smartphones and iDevices, your husband can follow along with your progress in a way that might have before been a little challenging.

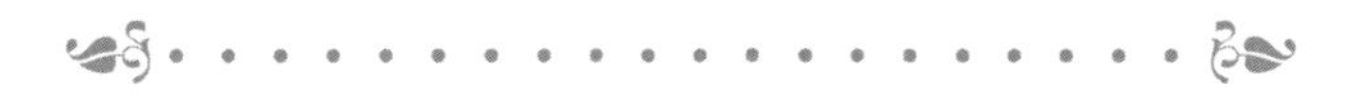

AS YOU CONTINUE ALONG THIS JOURNEY OF pregnancy, one of the things you'll note is how pregnancy resources describe your baby as looking "more human." I started to jot that down myself, for this book, when I realized that it's almost a silly thing to say.

On one hand, a three-week-old fetus doesn't look much like a just-born baby. On the other hand, they are both equally human, one imparted with just as much dignity as the other. That baby within you is certainly growing, however he looks! You know he's there, and your feelings are probably an unpredictable swirl. Do you find yourself facing special challenges or hurdles this week? Is there something you're holding close to your heart, an intention that weighs you down or fills you with worry?

Pregnant women have long held a special place in my prayers and my heart. There's something so amazing and intrinsically difficult about pregnancy that I keep track of people and make sure I pray for them in a special way when I know they're pregnant.

The dull aches and discomforts of pregnancy will continue to grow as your baby grows and your body stretches to accommodate its extra resident. Consider asking one or two trusted friends to pray for you in a special way during the remainder of your pregnancy.

TIPS FOR KEEPING DADDY INVOLVED:

- Involve Dad in assembling baby equipment.
- Take birthing classes together.
- Exercise together.
- Talk to him about how you're feeling at this stage in pregnancy, and keep the conversation going throughout the pregnancy.
- Invite him to your doctor appointments. Chances are he won't be able to come to all of them, but it will give him a chance to meet your medical provider, and it will give the two of you a context for pregnancy discussion, if you need one.
- If you're comfortable with him touching your growing belly, invite him to do so.
- Talk about your hopes and dreams for your baby, and imagine what the child's interactions will be with your current children.

Walking with Mary: The Crucifixion

It was dirty and uncomfortable at the foot of the Cross. She had endured watching him being tortured, and now, unbelievably, she was watching him die. I don't think, though, that she carried a heavier weight than I do when I weigh myself down with worries about what could happen, what might be, what's possible and probable, and potentially what's going to happen.

In fact, I wonder if there wasn't a certain freedom for Mary at the crucifixion. We know she had complete trust in God, so even there, at what seemed to be the end, she must never have lost sight of her faith and belief that God had it all under control.

I wish I could say the same. What keeps me from relying on God as Mary did? What stops me from letting God have my worries, my anxieties, and my fears? Why don't I just hang them up on the Cross with Jesus and let them die?

One Small Step

Every Catholic parish has a crucifix in it somewhere. I don't know how many times my confessor has given me the penance of praying before a crucifix for those who have wronged me or annoyed me. Jesus died for them, too, and he loves them just as much as he loves me.

This week, find a quiet half-hour to spend before a crucifix. Maybe it will be the crucifix in your house, or maybe it will be in your parish. Where it is isn't important. Focus on Jesus hanging there for all of humanity, and pray for that person or those people who you most need to forgive. Ask for the grace to embrace the love God has for you, and let it overflow into the rest of your life.

Faith Focus

Veneration of the Cross is a devotion that's most commonly held during Good Friday. As part of the communion service, everyone in the congregation comes forward, kneels, and kisses the cross (which is usually a crucifix). Our reverencing of the cross reminds us what happened on it.

I find it also reminds me what I'm called to do and who I'm supposed to be. When I'm having trouble sorting out my priorities, the cross stands before me, a litmus test of God's will for me.

Praying Your Pregnancy

Jesus, take the days where I wish I wasn't pregnant, and bless them with an awareness of how fortunate I am. Let me hold your mother's hand at the foot of the Cross and remain open to your will for my life. Amen.

CHAPTER 15

Week 19 (Fetal Age: 17 Weeks)

YOUR BABY IS GROWING AT A RAPID PACE, AND YOUR body is expanding to make room for the new life within it. You might not face worries during your pregnancy, and I encourage you, if that's the case, to spiritually adopt someone who does. Your prayers could make all the difference for her, and you might find, in the practice of praying in a committed way for someone else, that you are changed somehow.

Do you find yourself dizzy or light-headed at all? For me, this often happened because I would forget to eat regularly. I didn't become a good snacker until I was well into my first pregnancy. I'd have food, but it wouldn't be the kind that would really help me. I found that I needed high-protein foods to sustain me, foods like hard-boiled eggs, peanut butter, and yogurt.

During pregnancy, I found myself clinging to Mary's hand in a whole new way. When I had a particularly low day, I would think of how pregnancy must be in third-world countries, how suffering must be so much more poignant when you can't feed yourself.

Hold your sisters around the world close in your prayers. Use this time of pregnancy to unite yourself with Mary, and let her lead you closer to Jesus through prayer.

Walking with Mary: The Resurrection

I often wonder what it must have been like to receive the news that her son had risen. Did Mary leap up and dance around the room with a whoop and a hurrah? Was she immediately immersed in a prayer of thanksgiving, glorifying God for this unbelievable miracle?

We take the Resurrection for granted, I think, and finding the wonder of it takes a bit of work, at least for me. I need to really consider what death is, how permanent it is, the ways it wrenches every part of me. It is then, in the despair of facing death one-on-one, that the reality of the Resurrection can truly be appreciated.

Before I had children, figuring out how to die to myself was sidelined by my career, my prayer life, and my right-now life. Holding my first daughter, though, opened a part of me that I don't think existed before her birth. I learned that "dying to myself" involved putting others first, even at my own expense. This new approach required a different way of living. My natural selfishness became more apparent, and I learned that I needed to grow up in a lot of ways.

Motherhood has been a huge catalyst in helping me mature spiritually and emotionally. I have God to thank for this, and I look especially to the Resurrection as my model in motherhood. Every day, I have to die to myself—to my selfish inclinations and uncharitable tendencies—to take care of the small people God has put here for me.

Accepting God's will is not easy for me. I fight it so often, thinking that I know better. (When will I learn?) In the risen Christ, I see the effect of dying to myself: it is a glorious promise in the midst of the dirt and chaos of daily life. My struggles in the here and now are worth fighting, worth persevering, and worth continuing, when I look at the Blessed Mother and her son reunited outside the tomb.

Death has no hold over us. We are set free . . . if only we choose to be.

One Small Step

We recite the Creed—whether at Mass or as part of a devotion such as the Rosary—so often that we sometimes forget what we're saying. There's power in those words, and we proclaim them as the cornerstone of our belief.

The Resurrection is an important part of all of the creeds we use regularly in the Catholic Church. It's central to our beliefs as Christians.

Write the Creed—either the Nicene or the Apostles' Creed—longhand. As you write, pray the words with your whole being. Think of the impact of these words and of the meaning behind them. Let them soak into your mind and stay with you through the day. Hang the paper up where you'll see it, and repeat the prayer of the Creed at least once a day this week.

Faith Focus

The sacrament of Anointing of the Sick is typically employed in instances of grave illness or old age, but there are times during pregnancy when I think it's appropriate. One of those times, for me, is when I reach a state of worry that impacts me mentally.

Thanks to pregnancy, I have much more empathy for those around me who suffer physical limitations and ailments, and especially for those I know who are aging. It's because of pregnancy that I know what it is not to be able to sleep, and it's because of pregnancy that my body is a different place than it was before.

Anointing is a beautiful sacrament, and it may not be appropriate to ask for it for yourself. However, it is worth reading paragraph 1504 in the *Catechism*: "Often Jesus asks the sick to believe. He makes use of signs to heal: spittle and the laying on of hands, mud and washing. The sick try to touch him, 'for power came forth from him and healed them all.' And so in the sacraments Christ continues to 'touch' us in order to heal us."

At every Mass, we pray right before Communion, "Lord, I am not worthy that you should enter under my roof, but only say the word and my soul shall be healed." Healing is central to our human experience and our Catholic faith. We are all in need of it.

Consider your wounds, this week, and ask Christ to anoint you with himself. Open yourself to the healing that you need, and thank God for the chance to unite yourself closer to his son through the experience of your pregnancy.

Praying Your Pregnancy

As my body grows out and my baby gets bigger, God, help my love for you expand as well. Let me look to the risen Christ and see the glory of his wounds, even as I experience the many small humiliations of pregnancy and motherhood. Infuse me with the grace to believe the words I proclaim in the Creed and live them in even my smallest deeds. Amen.

CHAPTER 16

Week 20 (Fetal Age: 18 Weeks)

IT'S THE HALFWAY POINT. IS THE WORST BEHIND YOU . . . or ahead? I've been through pregnancy three times as of this writing, and I really can't answer that. For me, it depended on the day.

At week twenty, you might be past the morning sickness and well into the "feel better" part of pregnancy. You're probably showing just enough to make it clear to others that you're pregnant, but not enough that it's uncomfortable for you to stay active and involved in your life.

Your abdominal muscles are stretching as your baby grows and your body runs out of room and pushes outward.

Meanwhile, for your baby, a white paste called "vernix" is being released to coat your baby's skin, to protect it from the embryonic fluid.

At your doctor's visit this month, you'll likely have the opportunity to have an ultrasound, and you could even choose to find out the gender of your baby (or not).

By now, you might have a sense of your baby's acrobatic ability, especially when you try to rest. Does your baby respond to your voice, or to Daddy's voice, or to certain sounds?

It's possible that you're starting to feel a bit of "mommy brain" if you haven't already. Feeling fuzzy on details that you should know well, searching for a word, or forgetting things altogether, mommy brain is a well-documented phenomenon and lasts until you die. No, just kidding. Well, sort of.

Though your "old brain" may indeed come back, you will be changed enough by the new life within you that it won't quite be the same at all. You'll find a way to compensate and manage, and, I hope, laugh.

Walking with Mary: The Ascension

She looked up to see him leave. Was there a tinge of disappointment that she would be separated from him so soon?

As she looks up, she reminds us that heaven is our goal. We want to join her son there, with God, for all eternity.

When making it through the day is so much of a challenge, how can I think about heaven? Sometimes, I can only handle it one prayer at a time.

This week, consider how you can inspire heaven in those around you. It's so easy when I'm pregnant to become insular and forget all about those around me. I might still feed my family, but somehow it seems secondary to the work my body is doing.

At the Ascension, Mary reminds me to be mindful—despite serious episodes of mommy brain and frustrations. She looks up to the place where her son has gone, and helps me remember that my priorities are bigger than this life.

Try to remember those who are around you, even if it's as simple as saying a prayer for them—a Hail Mary, perhaps—when they come to mind or cross your path. As you find yourself frustrated, look heavenward and ask Mary to hold your hand and help you through your hurdle.

When the challenge of pregnancy feels like too much, ask Jesus to bless you with peace of heart. When the weight of your world is one ounce more than you think you can carry, ask Mary to point you to her son, whose Ascension reminds us that true beauty is attainable if we are true to the image we're to imitate.

One Small Step

I always know it's time for confession when I start becoming unreasonably annoyed with my husband. It's almost like I get a dose of mommy brain in my soul, and it manifests itself through my irrational irritations with my loved ones, and especially my husband. I made the mistake once of telling him this, and there was no blaming mommy brain for my mentioning this.

"How do I annoy you?" he wanted to know. I couldn't really answer well. The things that were getting under my skin were so small and forgivable that they didn't seem worth mentioning.

It's handy to have a built-in "radar" for confession. It's one of those things—like dental appointments and haircuts—for which I simply lack the motivation to schedule routinely. I find myself getting busy, and the first thing to be crossed off is that appointment I was supposed to keep.

I'm blessed with great teeth, and my hair can be tucked into a ponytail. When I start to let my spiritual life slide, though, everyone in my life feels it. I'm grouchy, I'm unfulfilled, and I'm hard to live with. Then I find little seeds of discontent sprouting into resentments and annoyances that are, upon closer inspection, very silly and inconsequential.

This week, make an appointment—and keep it—to go to confession. Then go a step further and make a follow-up appointment on your calendar. Now you're one ahead—in grace and in planning.

Faith Focus

"And behold, I am with you always, until the end of the age" (Mt 28:20).

Jesus reminds us that, though he has ascended to heaven, he is with us. As you face the last half of your pregnancy, turn your fears and worries over to his capable hands. Let him carry your burden and be your strength.

Praying Your Pregnancy

Lord, it's hard to believe I'm halfway through this pregnancy! Thank you for the gift of new life within and for the hope of life to come. Help me remember that the goal is heaven, and let me bless those around me by helping them get closer to you. Amen.

CHAPTER 17

Week 21 (Fetal Age: 19 Weeks)

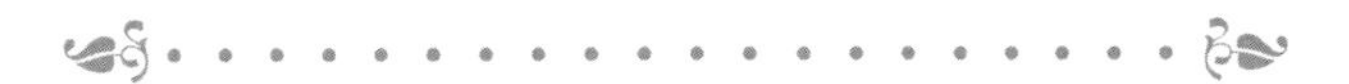

Coming to Terms with a Baby Who Might Not Live

By Jane Lebak

On February 28, 2000, my husband and I had an ultrasound to find out if we were going to have a boy or a girl. Instead we learned we were going to have an anencephalic.

If you've never thought of the ultrasound as a diagnostic test—if you've never thought of yourself as at-risk for a birth defect, it's worth the time to consider that doctors aren't performing them just to give Mom and Dad a photo for the scrapbook. They're looking for problems. And when they find one, many parents are put into moral territory they never considered.

Many parents are pressured to abort. The first doctor we saw, a doctor who lied to me and misrepresented my daughter's condition, pressured us to abort. I did my own research; I consulted other doctors. Abortion is immoral according to the Catholic Church even when the baby is going to die soon after birth. Well-meaning friends might tell you it's somehow "different," but it's not.

And so began twenty-two weeks of carrying a baby we knew would die shortly after birth. Time, it seemed, was a curse. The pregnancy was something to get over with.

Day by day, I realized I had a choice. I could blot out my daughter before she ever really lived, or instead I could treat this time as a gift. I could parent my daughter for only so long. How did God want me to use the gift of this time? How could I be a mother to Emily Rose as only I could?

I sang to her. I wrote letters. I bought things for her: things for the memory box and things for the casket. I prayed for her. I connected with other mothers, women who became my best support because they'd gotten through it. More than that: they'd become wonderful women. Maybe I could be a wonderful woman too.

It was the hardest thing I'd ever done: welcoming a baby I knew I'd have to let go, praying harder than I'd ever prayed in my life.

She was born one July night at 11:00 p.m. and died two hours later, at 1:00 a.m; a life measured in minutes and yet a life that changed our perspective, our marriage, and our understanding of children. I thanked God for the privilege of being Emily Rose's mother, and twelve years later, we still feel her impact on our family.

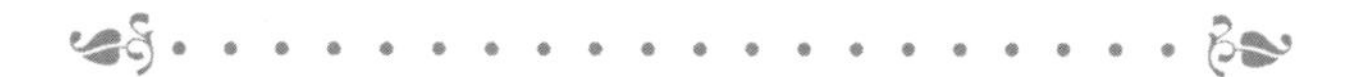

YOUR BABY IS ABOUT THE SIZE OF A LARGE EGGPLANT now, and he's hard at work swallowing amniotic fluid. This helps his digestive system as it continues to form and function.

While the baby's growth is slowing, yours is not. In fact, you might be experiencing swelling, especially in your lower legs, ankles, feet, and fingers.

You might also be well into the throes of experiencing a new approach to food. With my first pregnancy, I found, much to my horror, that I couldn't stand to drink coffee. I know coffee isn't a recommended drink for pregnant women, but I love coffee. It is one of my favorite things in life, so realizing that I couldn't stand it during my pregnancy shocked me a bit.

Each pregnancy is different, too. It's easy to be amused now, as I look back over my individual pregnancies and compare how they were different, especially in terms of food aversions. With my third pregnancy, I was able to drink coffee, and I consumed large quantities of certain name-brand packaged cookies. With my first pregnancy, I couldn't be near oranges, and I found myself sick the entire time I was pregnant.

Keeping some notes about the specifics of your pregnancy—including what foods you love and hate—is fun, because in five years, when you've forgotten the details, you'll be able to look back and remember things about being pregnant. And in five years that baby within you will be a rambunctious kindergartner who will be intrigued by the details of his time within you.

Walking with Mary: The Descent of the Holy Spirit

I remember bowing my head, sitting before the Lord in the Blessed Sacrament during adoration, and asking God to make me an instrument. I didn't really know what to pray or how to ask, but I had a strong desire to do his will, and I felt an urge, though I couldn't put it to words. I wanted to chart and plan, but I didn't know what I was supposed to do, so there was nothing to organize: there were no tasks or specifics.

All I could do was turn myself to Jesus. I always picture him sitting beside me with his arm around me when I'm at adoration. It's an intimate image, one where we are close and almost cuddling. I imagine that I can curl up beside him the way I do with my husband, and, in that comfortable position, confide the deepest parts of my heart.

For many years, the Holy Spirit has been difficult for me to grasp. He's without form, for one thing, so there's not a tangible or visual element. Picturing a dove descending upon me has always seemed sort of alarming. Fire above my head? Well, I have a bad relationship with fire after one raged through my apartment building in college, so that's not very comforting or inspiring.

It has taken me many years to understand the Holy Spirit in context of my Catholic faith, and it all started with that prayer during adoration. Jesus is a face, a human, someone I can approach. The Holy Spirit, though it has taken me longer to reach this understanding, is also a person, but he's a different kind of person—just as my children are vastly different (and yet eerily similar). So I have come to appreciate the third person of the Trinity in his own right.

The Holy Spirit was sent for each of us, to help us and guide us. He's like GPS, but with the volume turned way down. He will take us all the way to heaven, but we have to clear the clutter and clamor so that we can hear his still, small voice.

Mary is always leading us closer to her son, and she does it with the help of the Holy Spirit. She's the spouse of the Holy Spirit, which is a concept that helps me relate to the Holy Spirit. I understand spouses from my own experience with marriage. In fact, picturing the Holy Spirit as a tall, dark, protective guy like my husband, one who will gently carry me or fight through the difficulties to get to me, is far more helpful than the dove or fire images.

As your discomforts within your pregnancy increase, turn to the Holy Spirit. Ask him to bless this time that you and your child share in an intimate way. Hold Mary's hand and pray with her for the child within you to know the great gift of the Holy Spirit.

One Small Step

At Confirmation, we choose a patron saint and take that saint's name. This practice is to give us a model for our lives, one that will increase our practice of virtue and holiness. I think of having a patron saint as having a really good friend who you know won't steer you wrong. It's a way of stacking the deck in your favor.

The Holy Spirit is surely involved in this pairing, though I certainly thought I was the one picking my patron saint. As I've grown closer to the various patrons in my life—my own and my children's—I've come to appreciate how the Holy Spirit is at work behind the scenes. He moves so gently and quietly you might not even notice him. He's the breath of wind, not the loud wind or the earthquake (see 1 Kgs 19).

This week, turn to your Confirmation saint. Remind yourself of the reasons why you chose him or her initially, even if they're silly reasons. Explore the saint's life, and discover what more you have in common with this holy man or woman whose name you now share. Invoke your saint throughout the day, and ask him or her to lead you closer to God, especially the Holy Spirit, and to a greater acceptance of his will for you.

Faith Focus

"The moral life of Christians is sustained by the gifts of the Holy Spirit" (*CCC*, 1830). These gifts are wisdom, understanding, counsel, fortitude, knowledge, piety, and fear of the Lord. They "complete and perfect the virtues of those who receive them" (*CCC*, 1831).

When I look at that list of gifts, I can't help but smile. I know that the seed was sown at my Confirmation in my mid-twenties, before I was married or had any suspicion of someday being a mother, but I think it has been the crucible of motherhood that has made me lean into the Holy Spirit and depend on these gifts.

It's terrifying, looking at life and thinking ahead. I used to do it with a very goal-oriented mind-set, but now I try to approach it with my heart firmly in the Holy Spirit's hands and my hand firmly in Mama Mary's. I want to go where God wants me to be, but I don't necessarily need to know ahead of time. The reality of today—three kids, working from home, living in the country—would have seemed impossible to me fifteen years ago.

The gifts of the Holy Spirit bear some reflection, because I wouldn't have necessarily selected them if I were picking and choosing what I could receive. I might ask for patience or thriftiness as more practical applications, but I can see a bit how wisdom and understanding help me every day.

Consider the list of gifts and pick one or two. Examine them more closely this week, and think about their application to your life now and perhaps in the future.

Praying Your Pregnancy

Holy Spirit, fill me with the peace of your gifts. Inspire in me a passion for you and your will. Make me overflow with your love so that I may be a witness to those closest to me. Amen.

CHAPTER 18

Week 22
(Fetal Age: 20 Weeks)

YOUR BABY IS NOT MUCH BIGGER THAN A BANANA, and yet she has eyelids and eyebrows and even fingernails. She has details within you and is a complete little human. She has always been human, of course. There's something fun for me, though, amid the many aches and pains of pregnancy, to know about the tiny characteristics that are developing in the person within me that make her appear more human.

Your body is still changing. (Sense a theme?) If you're lucky, your sickness has passed and your abdomen, while enlarged, isn't so big as to hamper your movement. You might just be able to enjoy yourself and this pregnancy.

This is the point when I begin to feel the seed of excitement start to grow within me: I can't wait to meet the little person who punctuates my days with little fluttery kicks and rolls!

Walking with Mary: The Assumption of Mary

In the Assumption, we get a taste of flesh and blood. It's a mystery of the Rosary that, to me, blends the joy of family members all hugging each other with the brilliancy of great details.

Details make all the difference, don't they? Knowing that Mary was taken into heaven body and soul, showing Jesus's love for her—and for us—is a detail I can appreciate.

There are people I love who have died, some who are very dear to me. I can't wait to be reunited with them, to hold them in person, to share a meal, and to have all my favorite people in one place at the same time.

That's what the Assumption is: a gathering of all our favorite people—the saints, our loved ones, Mary, and God. There's food involved, and I think there will be hugging, too.

The Assumption also reminds me of my job as a mother, the goal of my vocation: getting to heaven those little ones I'm raising. It isn't easy and the job doesn't ever end. Someday, though, it will pay off, when we're all gathered together around the heavenly banquet, smiling and laughing in a way that's free from the burdens of this life.

IN THE UNITED STATES, WE ARE REQUIRED TO ATTEND MASS ON:

- The Solemnity of Mary, the Mother of God, on January 1
- The Ascension, which has been moved to Sunday from Thursday in many dioceses in the United States
- The Assumption of Mary on August 15
- All Saints Day on November 1
- The Solemnity of the Immaculate Conception on December 8
- Christmas on December 25

One Small Step

Chances are you will need to arrange things for your baby's Baptism well ahead of time. This week, in honor of the sacrament, make a list of what needs done to prepare for that joyous event, and complete as much as you can. If you need to meet with your priest, sign up for a class, or arrange the date, do your best to get these things done now. You'll be glad later that you took the time now to do them. Be sure to read part 3, and spend time prayerfully preparing yourself and making the necessary arrangements.

Our goal is heaven, and our "job" in our vocations as wives and mothers is to assist those in our care toward that goal.

Baptism is the first step. Don't underestimate the graces available to your child—and to you.

Faith Focus

According to the 1983 Code of Canon Law, Catholics are required to attend Mass and holy days of obligation. The holy days vary by country.

When most holy days—except Christmas—fall on a Monday or a Saturday, the obligation is removed. Our parish priest calls these non-obligatory holy days "holy days of opportunity."

Holy days do give us an opportunity to examine our faith and what we believe. Attending Mass—whether it's required or not—puts us in touch with the heavenly banquet in a tangible way. Find an appropriate reflection to read before or after you participate in Mass, and spend the day offering appropriate prayers related to the holy day.

Praying Your Pregnancy

Dear Lord, I know you must have a soft spot for mothers, because when I see how you lovingly took your own mother to heaven in the Assumption, I see a unique view of your tenderness. Embrace me with that tenderness this week, and guide me toward your loving arms. Amen.

CHAPTER 19

Week 23 (Fetal Age: 21 Weeks)

I REMEMBER PLAYING WITH DOLLS AS A GIRL, AND especially my Cabbage Patch, which I didn't receive until I was almost too old for dolls. I spent years wanting a Cabbage Patch—not a homemade one, mind you, but the real one, the one that came with the stamp on its butt and the box and the birth certificate.

A few years ago, my mom sent me a large box of things, and in that box was my Cabbage Patch doll. She looked very loved, and my girls, who had three of these between them before my oldest was five, were not very impressed by her. They were more intrigued by the many doll clothes my mom had made and somehow saved through the years.

Your baby's not quite the size of a Cabbage Patch doll this week, but he's close and weighs almost a pound. If you're feeling rounder, it's because you are. You've probably gained around thirteen pounds, give or take.

The difference between my old Cabbage Patch and your baby has to do with plumpness, and that's going to be the focus of his remaining time inside you: to add fat and weight to fill out his skin. He's going to fill out, and it won't be long before he's in your arms! Are you getting excited?

Speaking of excited, you might have noticed that people have one of two reactions to you: either a comment about how you're carrying twins or a question about whether you're really this far along, since you look so small. Oh, and did I mention mood swings? I probably don't need to: you probably know just what I'm talking about.

It gets better. Or rather, it gets different. (That's the story of motherhood, as far as I can tell.) Grip your Rosary and/or your favorite prayer card and practice your smile as you feel the tide of moods and comments sweep over you. Let go of your reactions and feelings to people's well-meaning (but perhaps inappropriate or ill-timed) comments, and embrace, instead, the love they intend to share with you during your pregnancy.

Walking with Mary: The Queenship of Mary

Time and three babies have softened me and continue to work on me. So does my relationship with Mary. I'm glad for this, and it's made me realize that yes, people can—and do—change. Thank God!

Now, mind you, I don't hear Mary talking to me any more than I hear God in anything other than a thought that comes out of nowhere. The voices in my head are, sadly, all me. But over the years that I've been Catholic, I have been drawn, over and over, to Mary. I've read about her and have prayed quite a few Rosaries.

As I feel myself growing closer to her, I find that Mary's coronation makes more sense. Jesus loved his mom so much that he gave her a crown. In my house of princesses and sparkly accessories, this is almost intuitive. A crown is almost a permanent bouquet to some people, though I think Mary likes her flowers fresh as much as the next mom.

My children do many things to show their love for me, and bringing me treasures is one of the most popular. These treasures might be drawings, favorite toys, or freshly picked dandelions. As I smile at them and enjoy their delight in sharing with me, I have an image of Jesus presenting his mother with a glorious crown, and I can imagine her pleasure. I think she accepts our little offerings with equal delight: we each bring her what we can with where we are in life. Her job is to help us grow closer to her son, who can equip us to give her even greater honor.

As you join the ranks of mothers—and maybe this isn't your first time, though adding a child always changes things—know that your relationship to Mary can blossom, if you let it.

One Small Step

A few years ago, I was at Mass early, which was a bit different than normal. Though my husband wasn't with me, my sister-in-law, mother-in-law, and two almost-teen nieces were, so the fact that I was the solo parent with my five-year-old and two-year-old wasn't so overwhelming.

I noticed, as we sat there, that the church was quiet, and then I realized that the woman who usually led the Rosary wasn't there. And with that realization, I knew something else without a doubt: I was supposed to do it.

Though I'm not scared to speak in public, I'll admit, right here, that I don't necessarily know the words to the Apostles' Creed, though I pray a daily Rosary (often using an mp3 downloaded version or an app on my iPad). I wasn't prepared for the adventure of leading the Rosary, but it had to be done.

It came out okay, though it turns out that I had started it later than I should have for Mass to begin on time at the pace I lead. We were just about to start the fourth decade when Father rang the bells to start Mass. (I'm comfortable enough with Father and my small country parish to just smile at this.) In his opening remarks, he told everyone they owed him two decades of the Rosary.

Consider leading a Rosary in your parish before a Mass. Make sure you ask your priest if it's okay with him, have written copies of the prayers in front of you, and have a support person there if it will help (someone you know will be nice about it and smile when you need it). Start with a daily Mass if you're very unsure of yourself. And, lacking a public Rosary, why not just ask the people who are there early to join you as you pray a Rosary quietly? You might be surprised at how many people will join in when they see you praying it.

Faith Focus

When I pray a Rosary, I think of it as putting a bouquet on my favorite mom's lap. It helps me to have this visual as I plod through it (it is never easy for me, no matter how often I pray it, and yet I feel I have to pray it). I'm taking flowers to Mama Mary, and if it's work to pick them or prune them or even propagate them, all the better for her. She knows the work I put into it, and she loves me for it.

I recently put in a few of my favorite plants on the side of my house, and they all have Marian ties. It's not quite a full-fledged Mary Garden, but I hope it will be someday. Why not research what plants you like that have Marian ties and create a Mary Garden of your own? It's a garden with extra meaning! You can get a start on learning more about Mary Gardens at the University of Dayton's Mary's Gardens website.[15]

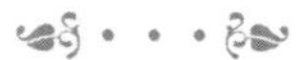

Praying Your Pregnancy

Jesus, I want to honor your mother, but sometimes it seems so theoretical. And, if I'm honest, praying the Rosary is difficult at best and harrowing at worst. Guide me to the time I need to sit at your feet, and put my hand in hers so that she'll lead me closer to you and your will for my life. Amen.

CHAPTER 20

Week 24 (Fetal Age: 22 Weeks)

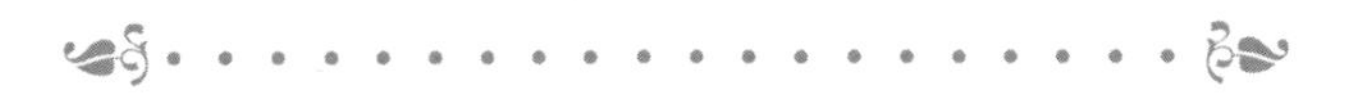

The Joy of Mothering Many

By Jennifer Fitz

"The baby is kicking. She hears you talking to her! She wants to meet you!" That's what I love most about the second, third, and later pregnancies: siblings. It's not just me and my husband waiting for this new little one, there's a whole family of other people to welcome her, take care of her, endure her colic, and videotape her first giggles.

My babies have a good PR team to be sure. "She's looking at you! She likes you! She's smiling! You taught her how to smile!" We do our part as parents to cultivate a friendship between siblings from the very beginning. But it isn't forced. Love is natural. It is normal for our children to want to love and to delight in being loved.

The first few months postpartum with just a newborn and toddler were my hardest ever as a parent. Labor, delivery, and newborn care were easier, since that was all familiar ground. But two little people who needed me constantly and in conflicting ways? Exhausting. Maddening. I couldn't possibly be everything they both needed. At one point I dropped them at their great-grandmother's in desperation, just to go sit and have silence for an hour.

The later babies were easier, because even a four- or six-year-old can provide some help with entertaining and tending to the toddler; it wasn't my first time parenting a toddler either. And friendships build so quickly. I remember my six-month-old sitting in the hallway, sounding yelps to summon her two-year-old brother to play with her.

My husband and I joke that each new pregnancy is a "promotion" for me—time to take my parenting skills to the next level. That's true. But it's also a whole new life for my other children as well: a new person, new relationships, new ways to help the family, new ways to share our home, new ways to play, and new joy for all of us.

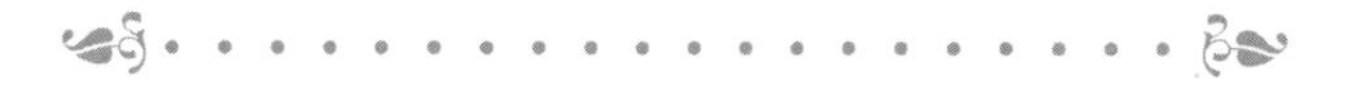

THINGS ARE GETTING A LITTLE TIGHT INSIDE OF YOU as your baby gets larger. She doesn't have the room to move as she did before, and you probably notice her cartwheels and gymnastics in a particular way.

As the time for your baby's birth grows closer, don't forget to reference sections two and three of this book. You want to be prepared for both labor and delivery and your baby's Baptism. Using the last half of pregnancy for your mental and spiritual preparation can be very fruitful—and it can take your mind off the anxiety that might be tugging at you.

Labor and delivery is a big unknown, especially if you've never been through it before. Though this is covered in more detail later in the book, I encourage you to begin working on releasing your fears. Let God carry them.

Are there other fears related to your baby that you've been harboring? Do you worry excessively about your health, your baby's health, your finances, your living situation, or something else? Do you find yourself anxious and unable to enjoy the anticipation of your baby's arrival? Is there something lurking, perhaps a long-overdue need for confession or a relationship you should mend? Make a list of your fears, and spend some time each day practicing giving them to God. You may not feel anything. It may seem fruitless. Don't give in to the temptation to give up, though. If this isn't a struggle you face at this point in your pregnancy, be thankful, and consider saying some prayers for those who do struggle.

. . .

This week in our Walking with Mary Rosary reflections we will start over with the first Joyful Mystery.

Walking with Mary: The Annunciation

Among Gabriel's first words to Mary were, "Do not be afraid." I wonder if she held on to those words as she reflected on the major life change resulting from her yes. I wonder if she remembered Gabriel's admonition months later, when the prospect of labor was looming, and life was looking uncertain as she traveled toward Bethlehem.

Was Mary scared? How did she battle her uncertainty and keep her trust in God? When did elation bubble over in spite of everything?

Gabriel's words are for each of us, too. Do not be afraid of God's plan for your life. Do not be afraid of the small blessing within you. Do not be afraid of what's ahead, but hold fast to God's hand, and use your will to choose to trust.

It's not easy to trust God, at least not for me. I want to be in control. I want to know what's coming and how and when and why. I long to run the show, but there is a great freedom in letting go. That's what trusting God so often is for me: letting go.

God has it all figured out, and he's far stronger than I am. By letting go—of my fear, of my worry, of my need to control—I free myself to do the important work that's right in front of me.

One Small Step

The word "vocation" still makes me think of "vocational education." During high school, I took classes in agriculture and was involved in FFA (which formerly stood for the Future Farmers of America). The purpose of vocational education—a phrase that has since been modernized to something else, I'm sure—was to train students for a trade. I was there because I wanted to be a veterinarian, and studying animal science is agricultural. I stayed because I became passionate about agriculture itself and especially the people.

I guess my adventure into my vocation as wife and mother wasn't so different, really. I joked, at first, that being married is considered a vocation because it is work. I stopped saying that, though, because it carries a negative connotation (at least coming from my mouth). It's true, though: marriage is work.

I was terrified to be a wife and a mother. I witnessed the pain of divorce firsthand and wasn't sure that marriage was worth anything anymore. I carried baggage, and no amount of theory or talking could convince me that I could do it. Though I still struggle with fear at times, I have discovered the joy of my vocation and the reasons it's more than just a job.

What makes the work of marriage and motherhood a vocation is the grace God sends to us, thanks to the sacraments. Whether you have a sacramental marriage or not, your reception of the Eucharist at Mass and your involvement with the other sacraments, going all the way back to your own Baptism and Confirmation, involve God and open your marriage to the opportunity for grace at work.

Now is a good time to stop and pay attention on purpose. What special graces do you receive as a result of your vocation as a wife? What do you have to be thankful for? What do you need to work on?

Offer the intentions of the next Mass you attend for your marriage. Hold the two-became-one that is you and your husband before Jesus, and pray for the grace to cooperate with all the graces available to you, thanks to your vocation.

Faith Focus

"Lord Jesus Christ, Son of God, have mercy on me, a sinner."

The Jesus Prayer comes from the Eastern Orthodox Church. It's one sentence, but it remains a powerful reminder for me. In those twelve words, my focus is turned to Jesus and to my need for his mercy. It's a call to action of sorts, in which I am forced to stop and realize that, if things are all about me, then I have a lot of work to do. Try punctuating your days this week with this short prayer.

• • •

Praying Your Pregnancy

Jesus, your mother heard the words, "Do not be afraid" when she was introduced to her vocation as your mother. Did she hear them again when she stood at the foot of the cross? Whisper them in my ear this week, and remind me to embrace the beauty in the many aspects of my vocations as wife and mother. Amen.

CHAPTER 21

Week 25 (Fetal Age: 23 Weeks)

IT'S HARD TO BELIEVE, BUT YOUR BABY HAS A VERY real chance of surviving if he were to be born now. There's always something freeing—and terrifying—about that fact for me. Up until this point in the pregnancy, he was sort of a theory . . . a theory that was beginning to kick and who made my life much different, but who was contained within me.

The idea of a baby in my arms, even after delivering previous babies, is always earthshattering to me. It shakes me up, and this is the week it begins to be real, the week when he could survive outside of me.

At this point in pregnancy, a prayer of mine always turns to "Let's make it to term, little guy," even when there is no indication that we won't. If I'm not careful, I find myself focusing on what-ifs and hypotheticals, which will only increase my blood pressure and cause me undue stress.

Have you started preparing your baby's "stuff" yet? The sheer volume always overwhelms me, and I find it a great opportunity to share with other women in my life. I'll sometimes invite my mother-in-law or a close friend who enjoys both organizing and baby paraphernalia to help me get things ready. Of course, twenty-five weeks is still early for that sort of thing, at least if you have any inclination to procrastination (and I do).

Walking with Mary: The Visitation

Imagine someone showing up today with a hot meal. Imagine, even further, if she stayed to clean up your house and help you with some of the more pain-in-the-neck tasks you haven't gotten around to lately.

You might not be completely uncomfortable yet, but you might find there are things slipping here and there. Add twenty years to your age, and you are, very likely, in Elizabeth's shoes. Then out of nowhere (because there wasn't texting back then), her young cousin showed up. I imagine them chatting away as Mary scrubbed her baseboards, dusted up her kitchen cupboards, or brewed her some tea (or whatever comfort drink they had in that day and time).

Mary might not have felt all that great early in her pregnancy, but she let her joy at Elizabeth's good news take precedence. I've felt that way before, and it's always a cleansing sort of experience. Doing something for others out of pure love, especially when I know it's appreciated, makes a part of me smile that needs to smile more often.

Women need each other, and most of all we need to have that camaraderie and community that we see so beautifully portrayed in the Visitation. Sometimes it takes a little letting go to invite someone in, to let him or her close to your heart. Maybe you don't know anyone who will bring you a hot meal or come and help you the way Mary helped Elizabeth. Look to the Visitation then, and see that every long journey—from here to heaven, from Nazareth to Judea—is made easier by having God for company.

Trusting God's will for your life isn't easy. In letting go of your plan, though, you open yourself to the wonderful surprise of Mary on your doorstep.

One Small Step

There are hungry people all around us. Many of them are hidden; the impoverished in my area of the country are camouflaged. Some people aren't hungry for food; they're hungry for love.

How can you show love to someone else this week? Is it by sacrificing an hour and praying before the Blessed Sacrament? Is it by preparing a meal or giving time at a food pantry? Give of yourself this week in some small way, beyond what you already do. It will be extra and it will be work. Make it a gift for Jesus.

Faith Focus

"The works of mercy are charitable actions by which we come to the aid of our neighbor in his spiritual and bodily necessities" (*CCC*, 2447). The catechism continues by listing both the spiritual works of mercy (instructing, advising, consoling, comforting, forgiving, and bearing wrongs patiently) and the corporal (physical) works of mercy (feeding the hungry, sheltering the homeless, clothing the naked, visiting the sick and imprisoned, and burying the dead).

We show charity—love—to our neighbor when we act in mercy, whether for the good of his soul or his body. Keep track of how often you act in one of these ways this week, and consider what you could do to make your actions more meaningful in this area.

Praying Your Pregnancy

Jesus, you were once the size of my baby. You inspired great things even before you were born—John the Baptist leapt inside Elizabeth, your mother Mary went in haste to serve her elderly cousin, and Joseph adopted you as his own. Give me the joy that was Mary's so that as I go into the final days of this pregnancy, I may act in love toward all those I meet. Amen.

CHAPTER 22

Week 26 (Fetal Age: 24 Weeks)

YOU ARE TWO-THIRDS OF THE WAY THROUGH YOUR pregnancy, and your baby's beginning to put on weight. You've probably noticed her active and resting cycles, and maybe she has been keeping you up at night with her gymnastics. This is part of her sleep-and-wake cycle.

Kind of hard to believe, isn't it? Your baby's just over two pounds and has her own circadian rhythm . . . while she's still inside you! It makes me want to stop and marvel and then stop some more and thank God.

By twenty-six weeks, your baby has all five senses fully developed. She can recognize your voice and might even react to it or to the voices of those around you. Both of my daughters had reactions to our priest's voice. I worked in the parish office during both of those pregnancies, and my oldest daughter would kick especially vigorously when she heard Father's distinctive laugh.

With each of my pregnancies, I gained insight into other parents. I spent time thinking of the poor women who felt that their only choice was abortion. I prayed for my own parents, especially the mother figures in my life—my actual mother and the many other women who have spiritually mothered me over the years.

Bringing another life into the world is a testament to hope, even if you don't think you have a lot of hope. It has taught me how hope and love are intertwined and how the seed of hope leads naturally to a blossoming of love.

Walking with Mary: The Nativity

The cave in Bethlehem probably isn't what Mary had in mind for her son's birth: straw as bedding and oxen as companions, with shepherds and townsfolk dropping in to wish her well.

After being told she would be the Mother of God, maybe she didn't find it that shocking that the birth didn't go at all how anyone would picture it. Even so, I'm sure it wasn't that comfortable even by standards of the day. She gave birth with animals all around, in the chill of winter, in a town far away from home.

So often, things don't go the way I plan. I struggle with my knee-jerk reaction to the wrenches in life, to the natural temper tantrum I want to throw. It's hard to see God at work in the up-close of a situation, turned differently from what I think it should be.

But he is at work. Jesus being born in the most humble of circumstances made him accessible to all of us. It also makes Mary someone we can all turn to for comfort: if anyone knows what it's like to go with the flow, it's Mary.

One Small Step

I thought I had all the details of my oldest daughter's Baptism planned to the hilt, nothing left undone. At the reception after Mass, though, our deacon walked up to me, cleared his throat and called everyone's attention to us. He then presented us with a lovely certificate, me with a rose, and my husband with a Rosary, a commemoration of our family's involvement in our child's Baptism. Our parish's Knights of Columbus council sponsors this for every baby baptized at our parish.

Not so long ago, my then three-year-old was crying in the night, scared of monsters. I handed her a Rosary and told her to hold Mama Mary's hand and know that her angel was there too, keeping the monsters at bay. The next morning, when I was in her room, I noticed that the Rosary she was sleeping with was one of the black Knights of Columbus Rosaries we'd received at these Baptismal presentations.

Pray a Rosary this week for a renewal in your own Baptismal faith. Ask Mary to guide you through the uncertainties ahead—both in the immediate future with labor and delivery and in the long-term future as you journey through your motherhood. Grab on to her hand, just as my four-year-old does every night, and trust that she will lead you right where you need to go, always closer to her son.

Faith Focus

The Angelus is a prayer that dates back to at least the fourteenth century. It is, essentially, three Hail Marys with a short verse in between, and is typically prayed in the morning, at noon, and in the evening. It's prayed in honor of the Incarnation, which is the act of God becoming man. If you don't know the verses and accompanying prayers (which are short), you can simply say five Hail Marys.

The Angelus Prayer

The Angel of the Lord declared to Mary:
And she conceived of the Holy Spirit.
Hail Mary, full of grace, the Lord is with thee; blessed art thou among women and blessed is the fruit of thy womb, Jesus. Holy Mary, Mother of God, pray for us sinners, now and at the hour of our death. Amen.
Behold the handmaid of the Lord: Be it done unto me according to Thy word.
Hail Mary . . .
And the Word was made Flesh: And dwelt among us.
Hail Mary . . .
Pray for us, O Holy Mother of God, that we may be made worthy of the promises of Christ.
Let us pray: Pour forth, we beseech Thee, O Lord, Thy grace into our hearts; that we, to whom the Incarnation of Christ, Thy Son, was made known by the message of an angel, may by His Passion and Cross be brought to

the glory of His Resurrection, through the same Christ Our Lord. Amen.

. . .

Praying Your Pregnancy

Jesus, you know how I feel about "going with the flow." As I journey closer to meeting this baby in person, hold us both close to your heart, and remind me that you have things under control, even when it seems like they are spinning crazily in all directions. Amen.

CHAPTER 23

Week 27 (Fetal Age: 25 Weeks)

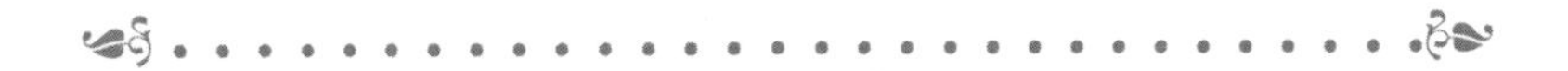

How Much Stuff Do You Really Need?

"You know, honey, you have enough clothing here for two babies," my grandma said gently as she folded and arranged things in the dresser before the birth of my second daughter.

I hadn't yet gone through my grand purging-and-reorganizing project that had me calculating exactly how many shirts one child really needed, so I bristled.

"Babies throw up a lot, and they go through a lot of clothes, and . . ." I replied. I'm sure I missed a meaningful glance between my grandma and mother-in-law, who made do just fine with a lot less.

When that second baby was just over a year old, I went through a decluttering process that had me giving away a lot of baby clothes. Our local pregnancy center and our younger siblings, who were having their own children by that time, were appreciative of the perfectly good clothing. And when I found out that I was pregnant with my third and that it was my first boy, I discovered that babies really don't need that much stuff.

Some of it depends on how often you do laundry, some of it depends on whether you need extra clothes for the babysitter or child care, and some of it depends on how much space you have.

I challenge you, though, not to give in to the urge to get every new gadget and baby toy. My babies have been just as happy with empty boxes as they have been with the light-up contraption from Fisher-Price®. Considering how fast babies grow, having fewer clothes will also leave you with less to pack up and put away.

WELCOME TO YOUR THIRD TRIMESTER. DOES IT FEEL like it came quickly? Do you feel like you've earned this? Just wait; the real prize is coming soon.

Your baby is adding length and weight and can now open his eyelids. His kicks also "count" now, and you probably have some ideas about his little personality from how he conducts his workouts within you. Maybe he's laid-back and just tickles you every so often or maybe he's a future tumbling superstar.

Are you thinking about who he will become, what's in store for him? Have you reflected on how his birth will change the world—not just your world but the world at large? What are your hopes and dreams, your fears and worries?

You might be counting kicks and starting to even think a bit about the reality of the baby coming out of there. In some cases, you might find yourself twiddling your thumbs in frustration from a prone position, assigned to bed rest and longing to feel productive again.

Whatever your state of mind this week, remember to stay positive. Don't let a snowball of helplessness—whether at the quick passage of time or the number of things to do—get to you. Turn your worries over to God . . . yell at him, shake your fist, and, above all, let go and worry no more. (Easier said than done, I know.)

Have you thought about whom you want with you in the delivery room? Some women want only their husband and possibly a coach or doula, along with any medical staff that may be involved. Other women invite parents and other people to be part of their delivery. Discern what's best for you and your husband. Will more people make more stress at a time when there's already enough stress, or will it be a way to share the miracle of birth with them?

Once you make your decision, stick by it. Don't cave in because you feel guilty. It's your baby's birth and there will be plenty of time to share the new baby once he's born.

Another thing to consider is who you'll call (or text, as the case may be) to let know that you're in labor and/or that the baby has been born. Coming up with a communications strategy, especially if you have older children, is easier now than later.

Walking with Mary: The Presentation

Jesus was the Son of God. He didn't really have to obey the law, because he was the lawgiver.

In the Presentation, where Joseph and Mary take Jesus to the Temple to be presented to the Lord, we see him doing just what he didn't have to do: obeying. It's a word that's not common anymore, and it certainly isn't popular (if it ever was). Being obedient is equated with being run over or brainwashed. It's not usually painted in a favorable way.

And yet, in the Presentation, we see Jesus's example of obedience through his parents. They committed him to God, even though they knew he was the Son of God.

In our own lives, obedience is often subtle, sometimes even invisible. It might mean skipping a fun night out because of a family obligation or not watching a show because of Mass. Obedience may include listening to the still, small voice of God in your life, or it could be eschewing something that leads you to sin.

What does obedience look like in your life? Examine it this week with the help of a spiritual friend or advisor. Look to Mary, and ask her for guidance.

One Small Step

Fridays are penitential, though we seem to have lost some of that in our cultural TGIF mentality. According to canon law, "the penitential days and times in the universal Church are every Friday of the whole year and the season of Lent" (1250), and "Abstinence from meat, or from some other food as determined by the Episcopal Conference, is to be observed on all Fridays, unless a solemnity should fall on a Friday" (1251).

For many years, I've done various fasts for my Friday penance. This week, fast from a favorite food or activity. Unite yourself with the Church and with God's will for your life and especially your vocation.

Faith Focus

The Chaplet of Divine Mercy was spread and promoted by Saint Maria Faustina and encouraged by Blessed Pope John Paul II. I discovered it as a new Catholic, and after I fumbled through it with the help of an audio CD, found myself turning to it whenever the weight of worry threatened to take over my mind.

Jesus's mercy is so great and so powerful that we should never hesitate to turn to him for help. Whether we're asking him to comfort us in what we think might be a silly fear or asking him to help us through another day of the same old stuff, he awaits our request with eagerness and enthusiasm.

When I don't know how to pray, or when the world feels too big for me to handle, or even when I'm just worried beyond my ability to deal with it, the Chaplet of Divine Mercy is the prayer I pray. When anger or frustration is eating me from the inside, it's the Chaplet of Divine Mercy that can calm me and focus me on my true priorities in life.

I have found that the time I commit to the Chaplet of Divine Mercy can be a penance that helps me grow closer to God and his mercy.

If you've never prayed the Chaplet of Divine Mercy, here's a short course using your Rosary beads:

- Begin with the Sign of the Cross, one Our Father, one Hail Mary, and the Apostles' Creed.
- On the first Our Father bead pray, "Eternal Father, I offer you the body and blood, soul and divinity of your dearly beloved Son, our Lord Jesus Christ, in atonement for our sins and those of the whole world."
- On each of the ten Hail Mary beads pray, "For the sake of his sorrowful passion, have mercy on us and on the whole world."
- Repeat for all five decades.
- Conclude by praying this three times: "Holy God, Holy Mighty One, Holy Immortal One, have mercy on us and on the whole world."

I have since discovered a sung version of this chaplet that helps me slow down while praying it. No matter how much I tend to "whip through" this prayer, especially when I'm most fretful, it never fails to remind me that God loves me and is just waiting to share his mercy with me.

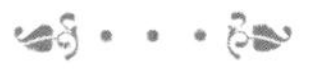

Praying Your Pregnancy

Why is it so hard to obey, God? Help me to be receptive to your law in my life; help me to obey in the best way possible. Amen.

CHAPTER 24

Week 28
(Fetal Age: 26 Weeks)

AT ABOUT THIS POINT IN PREGNANCY, THE SURFACE of your baby's developing brain—which looked smooth until now—forms grooves and indentations and the brain tissue continues to grow. Her hair's growing longer, too, and she's getting plumper. She now weighs around two-and-a-half pounds.

Have you noticed, as your pregnancy continues, that your tastes have changed? Foods you might have loved before might seem revolting, and you may find that you're eating things you never would have considered if you weren't pregnant.

Your baby's movements are now distinct enough that you can probably share them with others. Your husband, parents, older children, and friends may enjoy an opportunity to feel the baby's movements within you. And complete strangers in the store, noticing your belly, might feel the need to walk up to you and touch it.

There are times—many times—when I find myself cringing at loving touches, even from my children, and I have to sometimes consciously keep myself still so that they can tickle me or kiss me or even hug me. I have no idea why this is—I have no history of abuse or, really, of anything at all. It just seems to be how I'm made.

I didn't expect the sharing part of pregnancy, and I didn't anticipate the joy it would bring to others. Some women in my life—those who had already had children, mainly—seemed to identify with my state. And still others—especially my husband—were intrigued and shocked by the fact that another human being was inside me.

You are in a unique position: you are one and yet two. It's a responsibility and a gift, one that you can share with those around you.

Walking with Mary: Finding Jesus in the Temple

Can you imagine losing the Son of God? My reflections on finding Jesus in the Temple invariably lead me to imagine myself as the person who misplaced God. I imagine the head slapping and self-recrimination I'd be temped to impose upon myself and the hilarity I'd feel at finding Jesus right where I'd left him.

Mary and Joseph did not plan to leave Jesus in the Temple. He was supposed to be with the caravan. I wonder if they had a plan B for not being able to find Jesus in the caravan or with the stragglers in the back.

So often in life, I think I can plan my way to success. I have a plan A, and then I have a plan B. Every situation is covered, or so I think. Then reality hits, and it often looks nothing like what I've planned. I find, more often than not, that this is a good thing. It has taught me to trust in God and to believe that he really will be where I need him. Jesus doesn't need me to have a plan B . . . or even a plan A, much of the time. He simply needs me to trust in him and follow where he leads.

It's funny how something so simple—trust—can be so difficult. Mary and Joseph show me how to do it when I examine their finding Jesus in the Temple. They don't know where to look at first, but when they find him, they hold on to him. That's what I need to do, too: hold on to him.

One Small Step

I find Jesus in many places in my life. I find him in the people who seek assistance from our parish office, in the volunteers who are committed to helping within our parish, and in the friends and family members who show up just when I need them.

Think of a place you find Jesus—in your church, in a friend's home, in a favorite charity. Donate to that place as a way of thanking Jesus for being there. You might donate a monetary gift, but you could also perform an act of charity to help someone in that place. See how you find Jesus even more when you involve yourself.

Faith Focus

Saint Anthony of Padua is most popularly known as the patron of lost things, and I often joke that someday he'll help me find my mind. It can be no accident, though, that one year, in an online "have a saint picked for you" selection process, he was picked as my patron. That year, after I became pregnant with my second child, I learned that Saint Anthony is a patron of pregnant women.

He's a Doctor of the Church, and his teachings are simple and easy to understand. He was found, more than three hundred years after his death, with his tongue incorrupt, though his body had decayed.

In addition to being a patron of pregnant women, he's also a patron of women who struggle with infertility. Both of these are special intentions of mine and bring me closer to Saint Anthony. Turn to him this week, and ask him to help you through your difficult patches and keep you focused on the Lord.

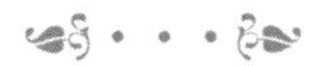

Praying Your Pregnancy

Where are you, Jesus, and why do you leave me here all alone? I need your help, but all I'm getting is static on the line! When I'm fumbling in the darkness, grab my hand and hold me close to you. Amen.

CHAPTER 25

Week 29 (Fetal Age: 27 Weeks)

YOU'VE BEEN PREGNANT LONG ENOUGH THAT YOU might be nice and uncomfortable. You might not be sleeping full nights, and you might feel like your bladder has shrunk to the size of a shot glass. The baby might have his own ideas about how you should sit, stand, or lie, and you might just be ready for this whole adventure known as pregnancy to be over.

Baby's not done growing, yet, and the next few weeks will help him gain important weight. These last few weeks are among the most challenging, though, especially if you are having increased difficulty moving and completing your normal routine.

It's okay to slow down. Whether or not you feel the urge to feather your nest, fold baby clothes and set up for your new infant, make sure you are resting enough. Rest does not mean, by the way, doing all your work sitting down, for example, while at your computer. (I need that reminder myself.)

Keep tabs on how you're feeling and whether your body might be sending you warning signals of preterm labor or complications. Ask for help—and accept help when it's offered.

Walking with Mary: Jesus's Baptism in the Jordan

Jesus didn't need to be baptized any more than he needed to be presented at the Temple when he was a baby, and yet he did get baptized. It was an act of humility, though I didn't fully appreciate it until I broke my arm on my thirtieth birthday.

There I was, with a two-year-old and a great deal of pain, with work still to do and no idea how I was going to get it done. At one point, I swallowed the hard lump in my throat that must have been my pride and sent an e-mail to a few close friends asking for help. I wasn't even sure how I needed help, but they were only waiting for the okay to come over. Within hours, I had a hot meal for my family, the leaning tower of dishes was being addressed, and a cheerful friend was insisting I lie down while her girls played with mine.

There's a lesson for moms of all stripes in this mystery. There's a great generosity in offering help, but it requires humility to accept help. There's a beauty in sharing our gifts with others, in offering and giving. There's an equal beauty, too, in letting others serve and in smiling and saying "thank-you."

There's no need for long explanations, for defenses, and for excuses. Look to Jesus in this mystery, and see the joy of the Father's approval. Look to John, and see the glory of the recognition of the Savior.

One Small Step

Priests and deacons serve so much in our parish communities, but they receive very little in the way of recognition. The priests and deacons I know eschew recognition and are usually first in line to shower others with praise and acknowledgment.

This week, find a way to show your appreciation for the priests and deacons who have impacted you. Recognize their hard work, the many sacrifices they make, and the invisibility that often cloaks their labor.

Faith Focus

There is a special service that comes through the vocation of motherhood, and I have found that some of the mother figures who have been the biggest inspiration in my life are those who adopted me spiritually. Some of these women don't have children of their own, but that didn't stop them from embracing their femininity and sharing it with me. Others have children of their own but have "adopted" me and continue to teach me, through their example, how the hard work I do in this vocation pays forward within the world.

Saint Anne was Mary's mother, and little is known about her. Tradition tells us that she bore Mary late in life. The Chaplet of Saint Anne is a beautiful devotion that calls upon the intercession of Mary's mother. This chaplet can draw me closer to the way the challenges of my vocation inevitably place me at Jesus's feet, if I let them. The image of a grandmother is one that is tender to me, and turning to Jesus's grandmother feels comfortable, homey, and cozy. I picture myself with a plate of chocolate chip cookies, fresh from the oven, peering up at a gray-haired woman wearing an apron and a welcoming smile, her arms just waiting to pat me or even hug me.

Pray one Our Father and five Hail Marys in honor of Jesus. After each of the Hail Marys, pray, "Jesus, Mary, and Saint Anne, grant the favor that I ask."

Pray one Our Father and five Hail Marys in honor of Mary. Pray, "Jesus, Mary, and Saint Anne, grant the favor that I ask" after each Hail Mary.

Pray one Our Father and five Hail Marys in honor of Saint Anne, following each Hail Mary with the same petition as before.

Praying Your Pregnancy

I'm uncomfortable, God, and I know there's a ways to go before this pregnancy is over. Give me the grace to accept the help I need and the humility to smile and recognize my own limitations. Amen.

CHAPTER 26

Week 30 (Fetal Age: 28 Weeks)

Naming Your Child

A name is important, and your baby's name is one of the most important responsibilities you have.

At least, that's how it always seemed to me.

Your baby's name . . . it's what you'll be whispering in the middle of the night, what you'll be shouting across the yard, and what you'll be hearing on the phone when someone wants to talk to her.

Do you have a family tradition you want to keep? Some people see naming as a chance to honor those in their lives; others see it as a way to set an example for the child (i.e., by naming her after a saint).

You might decide that you want to pick the name ahead of time and even, if you know the gender of your baby, begin calling your baby by that name while he's still in utero. I enjoyed being able to refer to my babies by name when they were still inside me—it made them more personal somehow, more tangible (as if the thumping in my ribs wasn't enough).

During my pregnancy with our oldest daughter, we called her by a nickname. When she was born, my husband and I were shocked—we wanted to call her by her full name, not the nickname. We have never called her "Beth" since her birth, in fact; she has always been "Elizabeth" to us. We didn't expect that, and I still find it amusing!

Would a rose smell as sweet if it were called by another name? I can't picture my kids being called by other names, but I don't really know the answer. I think that's a cue to us that naming is not a life-or-death issue. If you're not sure, consider praying to your baby's patron or to your patron saint for guidance.

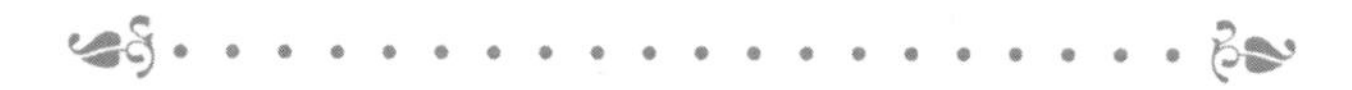

AT THIS POINT, I'M GUESSING YOU WANT TO HANG A sign on the inside of your uterus, declaring that you're out of room. You probably feel full in ways you either haven't experienced before or have forgotten. Maybe this pregnancy has been different from previous pregnancies, or maybe you are just done. Exhausted. Ready.

For me, this is the point at which I'm tempted to panic. Is there time to get everything done? (Never mind that "everything" is never done.) Will things go smoothly? (Never mind that "smoothly" is relative.) And could I please have another bite of whatever my favorite food is with this pregnancy? And a nap? And a foot massage?

I'd tell you to think about your birth plan, but the wisdom of the moms of many is that things will progress, despite your best plans. A plan can take you to a certain point, and it's a good place to start, but it's important to be open to how things go. You have to know what your priorities are for the birth, and chances are, you've thought about this a great deal during your pregnancy.

Your baby is growing and stretching you, and that's how motherhood is in so many ways. Whether this is your first baby or not, this child will change your life. You can plan for that, but probably for little else. The world is, in many ways, a great unknown right now, but you can rest assured that there is hope.

You represent hope. As you prepare for the exciting meeting with your baby, know that you are a beacon of the future as you give birth to a member of the next generation. Look past the discomfort, the inconvenience, and the pain. See instead the bright light of a child's understanding, the insight of a baby's laugh, and the sweet smell of a newborn's downy head. Ask for the grace to let go of your plans and embrace instead God's plans.

Walking with Mary: The Wedding at Cana

Two months before my wedding, my husband's brother got married. During the homily, our priest mentioned that the wedding, which was lovely, was only the beginning of a marriage. Marriage, he said, is so much more than the wedding day.

I've thought about that many times in the years since my own wedding day. I wasn't so keen to get married, just as I was very unsure about the whole prospect of being a mother.

Mary points us to the importance of our marriages at the wedding feast at Cana. There she intercedes for the couple when they've run out of wine, which in that day and time would have been socially catastrophic. She intercedes for each of us, too, in our marriages. On those difficult days and nights, ask Mary to guide you closer to Jesus. She cares about every single one of us, individually, and we should not hesitate to turn to her on our own behalf.

One Small Step

It's part of our vocation as wives and mothers to help our husbands and children get to heaven. Perhaps the most important way we can do this is to pray for them.

I discovered the power of praying for my husband quite by accident a few years into our marriage. Oh, I had heard about it, but to experience prayer at work was something else entirely.

My husband was miserable in his job, and I was feeling the effects of his misery. I felt like he didn't believe me when I told him he could get another position, despite his lack of a degree. A dear friend of mine encouraged me to pray a novena to Saint Joseph (and then she offered to join me in that novena). During that novena, my husband found out about a wonderful job opportunity, submitted a résumé, and was offered an interview. I began a novena in thanksgiving and our second daughter was born. While we were in the hospital for the two days following her birth, a message arrived offering him a second interview. He didn't hear that message until we were home with our baby.

He got that job, and I took the lesson to heart. My husband, to my knowledge, wasn't praying with me. I was praying for him.

Pray for your husband this week, in a concentrated, focused way. Ask him what he needs, and turn to God with that intention. Then step back and let God work.

Faith Focus

> "By reason of their state in life and of their order, [Christian spouses] have their own special gifts in the People of God." This grace proper to the sacrament of Matrimony is intended to perfect the couple's love and to strengthen their indissoluble unity. By this grace they "help one another to attain holiness in their married life and in welcoming and educating their children." (CCC, 1641)

Despite the dirty socks and hefty chores, though marriage is hard work a lot of the time and involves flawed human beings, we have a cushion of grace. Let's lean into that cushion and use it as much as we can.

Praying Your Pregnancy

God, you gave me the gift of my spouse, and I thank you for that. Help me to lean on him and trust him to support me in the last stages of my pregnancy. Give me the courage to ask for his help, the grace to pray for him always, and the faith to trust in the power of the sacrament that is our marriage. Amen.

CHAPTER 27

Week 31 (Fetal Age: 29 Weeks)

BABY'S STILL GROWING AND WEIGHS IN AROUND three-and-a-half pounds. You might be in the midst of crib setup, layette washing, and hyperactive nesting. My version of nesting was always to curl up with a book and convince myself I had plenty of time. At this point, you probably do, but it doesn't hurt to think about the basics, at least.

This is also the point of much swelling and extra saliva. Your feet may or may not still be comfortable in any shoes you previously wore, and your mouth may or may not be producing spit at a rate that leaves you drooling. You can thank the fact that your body makes up to 50 percent more blood and fluids during pregnancy. Your rings may not fit, and you may look at your extremities (the ones you can see, anyway) and wonder if you'll ever look the way you used to.

Well, yes and no. Yes, you will look non-pregnant again someday. No, you will not be the same as you were. Even if you return to your previous figure, bearing a child indelibly changes you. You could gain some stretch marks, which I've heard called a mother's beauty marks.

Don't roll your eyes at that: think about it and accept it, even if it makes you stretch mentally. God designed you to bear children, and that's what you are doing. Despite all the factors that should keep a baby from surviving in utero, you are nearing the end of your pregnancy. Praise God and thank him for the gift of your changed body.

And drink more water, avoid tight clothing, and don't cross your legs. That's supposed to help with the swelling.

Walking with Mary: The Proclamation of the Kingdom

I wonder if Mary appreciated knowing in advance that a sword would pierce her heart. I mean, it's sort of the state of motherhood, isn't it? You give birth (which isn't exactly a walk in the park), and then that little bundle of smell-good gets bigger and starts wiggling away in varying stages. Before you know it, you're waving good-bye as he gets on a bus, hugging him as he graduates from high school, and hiding your tears when he walks down an aisle to begin his own family or serve in some sort of religious life.

When Jesus proclaimed the kingdom, he wasn't necessarily telling people things they didn't already know. He was reminding them that following God is countercultural and that it takes work.

Have you ever had someone you love or someone you admire point out a major flaw of yours and make a suggestion for improvement? I've come a long way, because I no longer attack the person out loud when he or she does this. (I make no guarantees for mental conversations I might have with myself.) Over time, I've come to appreciate the tender voice calling me to change.

Jesus's voice in the proclamation of the kingdom is a call to each of us. He loves us more than anyone else, and that's part of the reason he calls us to repent and reform. He sees what we're capable of and how great we can be for God's glory, so he doesn't hesitate to encourage us. The path, though, isn't easy, and it involves swords in our hearts.

Jesus gently points us to the kingdom and he asks us to make ourselves humble enough to accept it. Can we do it? Will we say yes, just as Mary did?

One Small Step

Fr. Benedict Groeschel, in his audio reflection on the proclamation of the kingdom, states that the only place the kingdom can really come is in the human heart. To make room for the kingdom, though, we have to clear out the clutter of sin.

I have struggled for more than ten years with my spiritual director's encouragement that I go to confession regularly (he recommends at least monthly). I don't make a habit of mortal sins, and it's hard to make the time. Oh, and I have a lot of other good excuses too.

When I go to confession regularly, I find myself flirting with a feeling of the kingdom within me. Is that God's still, small voice amplified through all the empty space for the two minutes before I sin again? Could it be that I'm scrubbing off years of sin as I suck it up and go more frequently?

This week, go to confession, though you've probably gone recently (at least if you're following the "One Small Step" through this section). Dig down. You're probably "just" confessing "small stuff," and it might feel like nothing much. At least, that's what the devil would like you to think.

Faith Focus

I always expect a flogging after confession, but invariably, I'm assigned a prayer or act that requires me to get outside myself. In the *Catechism of the Catholic Church*, we're told,

> Christ instituted the sacrament of Penance for all sinful members of his Church: above all for those who, since Baptism, have fallen into grave sin, and have thus lost their Baptismal grace and wounded ecclesial communion. It is to them that the sacrament of Penance offers a new possibility to convert and to recover the grace of justification. The Fathers of the Church present this sacrament as "the second plank [of salvation] after the shipwreck which is the loss of grace." (1446)

Penance and confession are used interchangeably in many places, but I usually think of confession as the sacrament and penance as my assignment afterward, that which I have to do to make amends and show that I was serious.

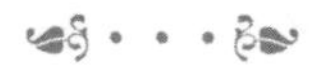

Praying Your Pregnancy

Jesus, I'm swollen and huge at this point, and as I look at my soul, I sometimes see that it's full of sin. Give me the grace to come to you and let you take it away from me. Fill me with love for you so that I don't want to stay away from the beauty of confession any longer than I have to. Amen.

CHAPTER 28

Week 32 (Fetal Age: 30 Weeks)

IF YOU'RE GOING TO A DOCTOR OR MIDWIFE, YOU'RE at the point where your appointments are increasing in frequency. Things are becoming more real, and it won't be long before you meet your little guy or gal face-to-face!

Be sure you ask your care provider the questions you think of in the middle of the night. Write them down so that you remember them, and don't be afraid of asking them. While you can probably Google or ask your mom-friends, I find it's a great help (and usually a comfort) to hear what my provider says about my question.

You might have reached the point where you find you can't do some of the things that you don't really want to ask help for, and this is the stage of pregnancy (which continues through the postpartum period, at least for me) where you learn humility in whole new ways. While I never actually asked my husband to shave my legs, I do know women who have. There were some things that I did have to swallow my self-sufficient pride about, though, like carrying heavier objects, dealing with bedtime for the older kids when I was just too exhausted, and even making dinner.

Asking for help is hard, though accepting help is even harder sometimes. We want to do it ourselves, which isn't so different from the behavior of a certain three-year-old I know well. There are things that are just plain annoying about pregnancy, but giving in to the urge to complain doesn't necessarily help. It may, instead, focus you in the wrong way.

I find it helpful to pick a psalm that's particularly poignant and read it out loud (and sometimes at top volume) as a prayer or pleading to God. Even better, write your own. Don't think that God doesn't care or that he doesn't want to hear. He does. In fact, the comfort he will give you will surpass the comfort of your best friend or spouse by a factor of infinite magnitude.

Walking with Mary: The Institution of the Eucharist

When Jesus instituted the Eucharist at the Last Supper, he began by doing what might have been the grossest act of service in his day: he washed the disciples' feet. During the Holy Thursday Mass of the Lord's Supper in our parish, our priest washes people's feet. Since our parish is small, it's open to whoever is willing to go to the front.

I've found, over the years, an interesting correlation. Kids are often enthusiastic about this and will be the first in line. Adults are less so, though some of them will participate.

In my own experience, I find it brings me to tears to have my priest wash my foot (which isn't nearly as stinky or gross as the disciples' feet were) and then kiss it. There's something tender and moving and, most of all, humbling about it. When I've talked to our priest about washing feet, he has said that it's probably his favorite act. He says it gives him a chance to say thank-you in a very personal way for the people who will allow him to wash their feet. He considers it to be a gift to him.

Performing gross tasks, things that people can't believe we would do for someone else, can be a blessing for them but also for us. It's a two-way street of blessing, and when we avoid either end of the equation, we lose—or keep someone else from losing—the blessing that's waiting for us.

When can I say yes to someone else's offer? How can I embrace the service for me and return it in a way that will make me a channel for God's grace? In an act as simple—and as disgusting—as washing feet, Jesus inspires each of us to give until it hurts.

One Small Step

Each of us has a vocation. Your vocation as a wife came about because of the sacrament of Matrimony. Some are called to the single life, others to the priesthood or diaconate, and still others to consecrated religious life. When we pray for vocations, we often neglect to pray for them all.

It's common to hear about a priest shortage, especially here in the United States. However, I think we should pay attention to the shortage we have of strong marriages and the support we seem to be losing when we embrace our feminine dignity, expressed as wives and mothers.

We, too, serve. We, too, pray. We, too, have a vocation, and it's one that is vital and much needed in today's world. We have an opportunity to serve with every diaper we change and every load of laundry we do. We imitate Jesus and let him shine through us when we not only perform these acts but also turn them into acts of love.

This week, make a point to pray for vocations—all vocations—every day as you do your most disgusting duties. If you attend an extra Mass, offer it for an increase in holy vocations.

Faith Focus

> The word "ordination" is reserved for the sacramental act which integrates a man into the order of bishops, presbyters, or deacons, and goes beyond a simple election, designation, delegation, or institution by the community, for it confers a gift of the Holy Spirit that permits the exercise of a "sacred power" (*sacra potestas*) which can come only from Christ himself through his Church. Ordination is also called consecratio, for it is a setting apart and an investiture by Christ himself for his Church. The laying on of hands by the bishop, with the consecratory prayer, constitutes the visible sign of this ordination. (CCC, 1538)

We aren't ordained into our roles as wives and mothers the same way these men are ordained into their vocation, but we can learn from their lives of service and sacrifice. We choose our vocations in different ways, but we are all united in the Body of Christ. Learn more about your priest or bishop as a man, and find a way to help him from your corner of the world, whether in prayer or service.

• • •

Praying Your Pregnancy

Lord, bless my vocation as wife and prepare me for your many graces as I begin a new phase in my vocation as a mother. Amen.

CHAPTER 29

Week 33 (Fetal Age: 31 Weeks)

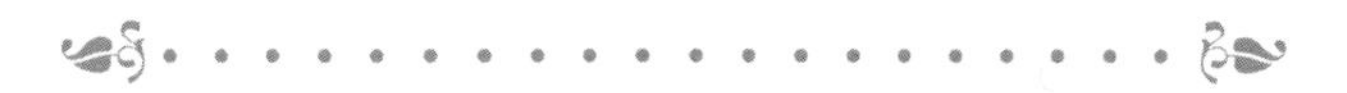

Finding Peace in Stillbirth

By Karen Murphy Corr

I cannot articulate the indescribable agony of realizing that your infant has died. Of having to inform the older siblings that their baby is not coming home to grow up with them. Of watching the older siblings hold their baby brother's body and come to terms with the concept of death. Of having to plan a funeral Mass. Of dealing with milk coming in when there is no baby to feed. Of dealing with the well-meaning comments from family and friends who want to stop your pain and in so doing deny your grief and want to rush you back to happiness and normal when life is anything but normal. Of feeling like a walking worst-case scenario and having no one want to believe that in this day and age healthy babies die. Of learning how to answer the question about how many children you have without falling apart.

Stillbirth is more than four times more common than Sudden Infant Death Syndrome (SIDS), but no one accepts statistics on modern infant mortality until she is part of the sad sorority. People want to believe there is a reason why babies die, and they grow impatient with a woman who is "still" sad just weeks after her baby has died. I had to point out again and again that I was a postpartum mother with all of the hormones and none of the perks.

Seeking out other bereaved mothers online was a huge support, as was meeting other baby-lost mothers in real life. Morning Light Ministry, a Catholic ministry, was a huge comfort, as was the chapter on stillbirth and pregnancy loss in Kimberly Hahn's book, *Life-Giving Love: Embracing God's Beautiful Design for Marriage*. A huge challenge was deciding whether my heart could handle being open to another pregnancy now that I no longer felt a healthy pregnancy would necessarily result in a living baby to bring home. I have a small prayer book by A. Francis Coomes, S.J., called *Mothers' Manual* that has beautiful prayers for bereaved mothers. I read them over and over, praying them when I felt too empty to pray otherwise. I meditated on the agony and passion of our Lord and the undoubted agony of Our Lady as she watched her son die. They knew agony and loss.

On March 7, 2011, I gave birth to our sixth child. I didn't broadcast news that we were pregnant until we had to, and I could not count on a healthy, happy delivery for my own sanity. I prayed a novena to Saint Gerard, but still prepared myself that this baby might die as well. The healthy, happy arrival of baby Margaret has been healing for our family, but our delight in her wriggly, happy little self does not lessen our sorrow in losing George. Losing a child means living incomplete until that day we are all reunited for eternity.

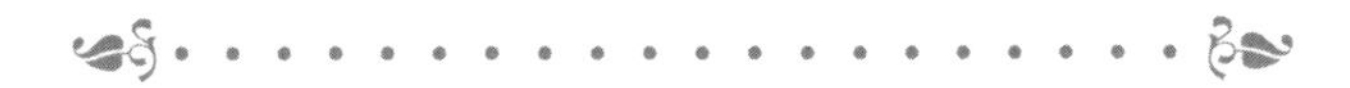

YOU'VE MADE IT ANOTHER WEEK CLOSER TO MEETING your baby. Congratulations.

You are growing a human being and, in this final stretch, it feels like work, doesn't it? Rest. Take a nap. Read a book. Rest some more. You're probably waking at least once through the night, and though some would tell you that's preparation for when baby comes, I'll tell you that it justifies a nap during the day.

Sleep is highly underrated, but you need it now and after the baby's born. It took me a few years and two babies to realize that I was ignoring my body's most important need when I burned myself out again and again. When I reached depression stage a year after my second child was born, I started looking for clues and things that fed my depression.

I was shocked to find that sleep topped the list. When I'm sleep deprived, things seem impossible, and my level of negativity shoots to the sky. In the midst of it, I will think I'm being completely calm and rational, but when I look back, I realize that I was anything but. It's hard to deal with the day-to-day hilarity and adventure when I'm tired.

I find, though, that I can't nap very well. I have to be completely exhausted to consider it, and then I don't fall asleep easily. Initially I thought this meant that I just had to keep going. I've learned, though, that it means I need to find a way to rest and, if possible, talk myself into sleeping, even if it is daytime and I feel like I'm missing out on life.

Prior to having my second child, my motto was "I'll sleep when I'm dead." There have never been enough hours in any given day for me to do all I want to do, and accepting that sleep—like food—is not optional was a journey for me. I share it here in the hope that you can take it to heart and put it at the top of your priority list before you suffer any ill effects.

Life with kids doesn't always allow sleep, and there are seasons when there's not time for much else besides sleep. Know that it shall pass, it will get better, and you will walk out into the light of a new season of your motherhood.

Walking with Mary: The Agony in the Garden

I think Jesus' time in the Garden of Gethsemane must have been a special kind of horror. He knew what was going to happen—he saw it coming, but he was powerless to stop it. "Not my will, but Your will, Father." He sweated blood.

If you had told me, hours before my five-year-old daughter had her first stroke-like seizure, that I would face that situation, I think the dread of it would have been far worse than the actuality. It was pretty bad, don't get me wrong, and I rank it as one of the worst experiences of my life. My husband has said since that nothing can really scare him now. "I held my baby and didn't know if she would make it," he said. "The drama at work just doesn't get me riled."

There is a gift in not knowing what's coming. It makes me look to this mystery with even more compassion for Jesus. Poor guy, he saw it coming. He knew what would happen. And, perhaps because of the example of his mother for his whole life, he said yes.

God's will. I don't understand it in the moment. I don't even usually want to do it. But when I do—when I let go and embrace the gift of his roadmap—I find that he equips me for far more than I could have imagined on my own.

One Small Step

You are probably anticipating labor and delivery at this point, and you might have conflicting emotions. If this is your first baby, you are facing a great unknown. If this is a subsequent baby, you might be more confident . . . and yet, there's that old maxim that every baby is different.

You're big and swollen and miserable, to some extent. This week, make something beautiful, and make yourself beautiful too. Wear lip gloss, style your hair with extra care, and add some jewelry. Maybe you can splurge and get your nails done or have your hair trimmed and styled at a salon. Be pretty and enjoy it. Your body, however misshapen and full of baby, is a temple of the Holy Spirit.

Faith Focus

There's holy water at church, but did you know you may keep holy water at home too, and bless yourself with it? All you need to do is take a clean container to your parish church and look for a faucet labeled "holy water." (If there isn't one, talk to your parish office or even your priest.) Since there's no cost to the "making" of holy water, there's no expectation of an offering in return.

You might keep it in containers at home, or you might have a font of some sort at your house. Some people travel with holy water (even in their car just to run errands), and others just use it at church.

Praying Your Pregnancy

Dear Jesus, walk with me in these final weeks of pregnancy, and hold me close to your Sacred Heart. I am looking forward to meeting this baby, but I'm not necessarily looking forward to the process that gets me there. Keep me wise as I prioritize and focus always on God's will for my every day. Amen.

CHAPTER 30

Week 34 (Fetal Age: 32 Weeks)

YOU'RE ABOUT TO EXPLODE WITH ANOTHER PERSON and, well, it's just plain uncomfortable. That is okay. It's common. You're not a freak.

You're doing a great job. I don't care if you've gained twice as much as the doctor said you should or if you feel like a total failure. I want you to look in the mirror and picture the woman God wants you to be. Now, today, be that woman. You'll need his help. Lean on him.

You can do this. There's not much left, and I'll be encouraging you in the next section, too, but it doesn't hurt to hear encouragement while you're ready to burst.

I've never run a real race, like a 5K, but I remember being in gym class and watching runners in the Olympics and track teams. At the end of a long, grueling race, somehow they had it in them to sprint. I'm not that person. I am the one crawling, stumbling, and only refraining from loud howling due to a shortage of oxygen in my system.

At this point in pregnancy, I always feel like I should be embracing things with a smile when what I want to do is chuck it all over my shoulder. Though I picture the many women I know who long for children and feel guilty about my hatred of my discomfort, each day I have to face where I am. That's where God meets me: where I am, not where I'd like to be.

I'd like to appreciate my blessings, but sometimes blessings are hard work. Sometimes blessings drain all my energy, keep me from sleeping, and are way different in practice than they were in theory.

Being pregnant is, above everything else, a blessing. That doesn't make it easy or comfortable, though, and it gives you room for reflection. Reflecting might be the last thing you feel like doing, but I encourage you to consider it. Make a quiet space in your week and sit at Jesus's feet. Give him your discomfort, your fears, and even your joy and anticipation. You don't have to do this alone!

Walking with Mary: The Scourging at the Pillar

There's no doubt it was painful to be scourged. Jesus's flesh was torn by the shards on the end of the whips.

Picture the people observing. There's no reason to suspect the Romans would have had any fondness for him, but in the crowd of leering, goading people, there had to be people who had listened to Jesus's preaching. There must have been people who were close to him, who had even cheered him on in his ministry and encouraged his miracles. It's possible that his mother was there, too, seeing her son ripped to shreds.

What must it have felt like to see those people laughing and even enjoying the scourging? How must Jesus have felt in their betrayal? How much more did it hurt, knowing his mother—who had also done no wrong—was suffering as she watched (or would suffer later while seeing him)?

We've all experienced betrayal. There's a special sting when we find out that someone who seemed to be our number-one fan maybe isn't so much or seems to have changed his or her mind. There's also a prick I often give myself, thinking that I know what someone else thinks of me. I'll get myself all worked up, thinking that Joanna believes I'm a total idiot about the decision I made (and am standing by).

Is it worse to be betrayed or to be flogged for something we didn't do? I change my mind on this, depending on the day.

The lesson in this mystery is one that I need: Jesus understands. Oh boy, does he understand. Maybe he wasn't ever pregnant with his fourth kid and up to his ears in housework and feeling the pressure of a distant family member to come visit as soon as the baby's born. Having gone through the exact scenario isn't necessarily a prerequisite for being able to understand though. Can't you picture his pain and torture in this mystery? Can't you imagine, to some extent, the horror and weight of it?

Turn to Jesus, in this mystery, and tell him about what scourges you. Give him the heaviest burden you have, the one you think he will least understand. Use this mystery as your common ground, as the place where you meet him. Let him guide you to the place of blessing, where the pain might make sense or have a purpose, perhaps even eternally.

One Small Step

There's a psychological concept, my brilliant doctoral-level social scientist sister-in-law assures me, in which it's easier to like someone who you think likes you. The reverse of that is also true: it's harder to like someone who you don't think likes you. The key word here is "think."

This week, encourage someone who you think doesn't like you. You might send a small note or even make the person a meal. You don't have to go overboard—this is a small step, after all.

Faith Focus

The scapular is, technically, part of a monk's garb. It's been adapted over the years into something that many others wear. The most popular ones look like two small squares of cloth attached by string, so that the entire thing makes a circle.

The most popular scapular, the brown scapular, is a result of an apparition of Mary telling Saint Simon Stock to wear it in 1251. It was to be a sign of salvation, as well as a protection and pledge.

Wearing a scapular can have privileges and indulgences attached to it, but I wear one at times for two different reasons. First, when I fight fear and anxiety, I find that nothing reminds me of my safety in God's arms like having a scapular around my neck. Second, a scapular around my neck is a tangible reminder of my faith. Though there are a lot of other ways I can remind myself, the slight movement of one of the pieces of cloth, the scratchy feeling of it getting caught in a necklace, and my kids pulling it out of my shirt to examine it all stop me and remind me where my priorities should be.

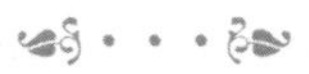

Praying Your Pregnancy

Dear Lord, how can I still have more than one week to go? Guide me, as I feel so conflicted about life in so many ways, and help me to remember your deep love for me. Amen.

CHAPTER 31

Week 35 (Fetal Age: 33 Weeks)

'TIS THE SEASON OF BRAXTON HICKS AND DROPPING babies, and these are indications that you are in the home-stretch. Things are so different now, you might not even recognize yourself. Are you trying not to laugh too hard or sneeze or cough? (If you don't know why I'm asking, then count yourself better at Kegels than I ever was.)

Have you talked to your husband about his role in your labor and delivery? If not, make some time to start the discussion, and begin thinking about it together. It's not possible to foresee how labor will go, but if you feel unsure, consider that your husband feels about ten times more unsure than you—it's not his body, after all.

Walking with Mary: Crowning with Thorns

She held that head, cradled it against her breast. She stroked the downy hair in his infancy, kissed his forehead during his boyhood, and watched it change and mature.

Seeing it streaked with blood and torn apart by the thorns must have been especially surreal for Mary. He was her baby, and yet he wasn't hers at all.

I think of this mystery when I face challenges—especially of the health variety—with my own children. My worries about their well-being and even survival are trumped by the knowledge that they're not really mine at all: they are God's. They are merely given to me in trust, for a time. Only God knows how long I will have them to hold here on earth, and accepting that with a smile is one of the hardest parts of my vocation as a mother.

Can I give my child back to God, with a willing heart? Will I accept God's will and his design for my life and the life of my children? How can I hold Mary's hand and place my trust at her son's feet with regard to my children's well-being?

Mary knows our struggles. She saw her child suffer, and instead of letting herself become bitter or enslaved to the better future she could have imagined, she let God lead her. Can I let God lead me to the joy of his plan?

One Small Step

Spiritual adoption is the practice of adopting someone through your prayers. You might make sacrifices for their intentions or pray intentionally for them each day. It can vary widely in practice, but the heart of it is having someone specific in mind and offering your prayers and other sacrifices for him or her.

This week, spiritually adopt someone who's recently been confirmed. It might be a young person in your parish or an adult. It could be someone who's been confirmed in the last year or in the last month: you decide. Begin a novena to the Holy Spirit (which can be as simple as praying the "Come Holy Spirit" prayer every day for nine days) for the person and his or her growth in holiness.

Faith Focus

Our Lady of La Leche is a title of Mary's that might have originated because of the Milk Grotto in Bethlehem. According to tradition, Mary and Joseph stopped there to hide during King Herod's slaughter of the innocent male children. Tradition holds that Mary nursed Jesus here, and a drop of her milk hit the cave's floor, making the rock white and chalky. Women now mix a bit of this dust with their drinks to help increase fertility and milk production.

You don't have to travel to Bethlehem to have a conversation with Our Lady of La Leche, though. Think of Mary performing actions similar to what many women do with their babies and what you will do so soon with your own baby. She becomes more real, more accessible, and more human—and so does her son.

As Our Lady of La Leche, Mary holds a nursing infant and smiles at each of us, whether we find ourselves longing to hold our infant or to take a break from the fray our children place in front of us.

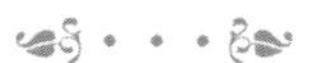

Praying Your Pregnancy

I feel so close, and yet so far away, Jesus. There's so much left to do. And yet, I can't wait to hold this baby in my arms. Give me patience with those around me and with myself. Guide me to your arms when I'm most frustrated with the challenge of the day. Amen.

CHAPTER 32

Week 36 (Fetal Age: 34 Weeks)

AT THIS POINT IN PREGNANCY, WITH ONLY FOUR OR five weeks until your due date, your amniotic fluid levels have peaked. Your baby will keep growing, though, and your body will reabsorb a bit of the fluid. That means your baby's space within you is becoming cozier. His movements may feel a little different to you as a result, or he may move less.

With my third pregnancy, around this week, a certain member of my family started asking me—daily, it seemed—if I had my bag packed for the hospital. I laughed every time she asked. I often replied with, "Come on! I'm on my third pregnancy. It doesn't just happen in a boom. There will be no rushing to the hospital! Besides, I have weeks to figure that out."

As it turns out, we were both right. Thanks to her insistence, I did have a bag ready when I had to go to the hospital a few weeks later in a bit of an unexpected hurry. My confidence that I had "been there, done that" meant that I had a list on top of the packed bag, with a reminder of what needed shoved in at the last minute, including (but not limited to) my husband's iPod touch, my laptop, and at least two of my current reads, because with our second delivery we found ourselves bored for a big chunk of time. (Shake your head at me. I know.)

You probably don't need your bag packed yet, but it might help to think about what you'll want to take. It will save your husband a trip home to get what you could have had ready but forgot as you left the house.

Walking with Mary: Carrying the Cross

It's heavy, it's annoying, and it's unwanted. Whether it's a sick child, a fussy baby, or a load of pukey laundry, it's a cross. It might be a chronic pain or illness, the suffering of a loved one, or a situation you have to endure. Whatever your cross is—the constant cross and the current cross—it's not easy to carry.

As Jesus stumbled with his Cross, there was a chorus of scorn coming from the sidelines, mingled with the howls of mourning women. Sweat was running down his body, stinging the freshly opened cuts.

With each step he took, he was closer to the glory that would come through the Cross. No one else saw it—though Mary must have seen it—as God's will. She said yes as she stood there, mute in the face of the horror. She accepted God's will, even as she wondered why and how.

We each carry our own cross, but we are not alone. At this point in pregnancy, your cross might be inside you, but you are not alone. Whether or not you have a network of family and friends, you have a heavenly Father and a host of saints who are praying for you.

One Small Step

Motherhood has been the best classroom for me for learning what "dying to self" truly means. There are many opportunities to succeed—and fail—each day (for that matter, each hour).

This week, examine how you might die to self in your everyday interactions. Each day consciously die to self with some action or sacrifice or prayer.

Faith Focus

The Via Matris or Way of the Mother is a devotion brought to us by the Servite Order. It's a set of seven stations observing the seven sorrows of Our Lady. At each station, reflect on Mary's sorrow. After reflecting on the station, pray a Hail Mary and "Mother, Most Sorrowful, pray for us."

1. Simeon's prophesy that a sword would piece Mary's soul
2. Joseph and Mary fleeing with Jesus into Egypt
3. Mary and Joseph searching for Jesus in the Temple
4. Mary meeting Jesus as he carries his Cross on the way to Calvary
5. Jesus dying on the Cross
6. Mary receiving Jesus's body in her arms
7. Jesus being laid in the tomb

After you've reflected on all the stations, end with three Hail Marys.

• • •

Praying Your Pregnancy

I want to be ready, God, but I feel like I could be taken by surprise at any moment. Give me peace of heart and the grace to cooperate with your will today. Help me to carry myself with the joy of knowing you are by my side. Amen.

CHAPTER 33

Week 37 (Fetal Age: 35 Weeks)

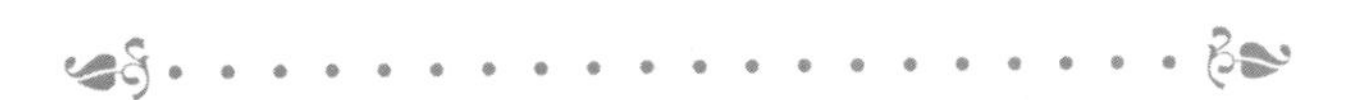

When Labor Doesn't Go as Expected

By Dorian Speed

We're now three for three with babies going to the Neonatal Intensive Care Unit (NICU) right after delivery. We joke that it's our own version of going through Customs, but of course it's been quite stressful. I don't even know what it's like to be handed my baby after giving birth, since each of mine has been whisked away to intensive care.

When my oldest was born, I had to have an emergency C-section, which came at the end of a long, difficult, and not-according-to-plan labor. We'd taken classes and done everything we could to ensure a natural delivery, but it wasn't to be—even our doula attested that a surgical birth was the best possible outcome. And I am very grateful for the skillful hands of the surgeons who brought each of my children into the world.

When things don't go as you've hoped, it can be tempting to retrace your steps and to wonder if you could have made other choices along the way that would have produced a better outcome. Give yourself permission to feel sadness along with the joy of meeting your new baby, but don't entertain thoughts of what you could have done differently.

While I've sat by the bedsides of my babies, peering past the tubes and cords, the image of Mary and Elizabeth rejoicing in one another's pregnancies has brought me great comfort. We have been fortunate to have wonderful support from friends and family who prayed, cooked, and ran errands. These generous offerings have reminded me to be grateful even when our joy was tinged with suffering.

There is silence amid the beeping and intercom announcements in the hospital, a restful silence perfect for prayer and contemplating the beauty of your newborn child. Let your heart be at peace, come what may, and know that you and your baby are never alone.

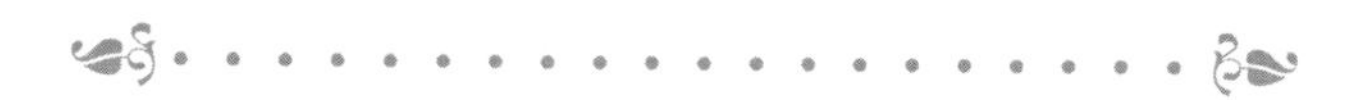

AT THIS POINT, YOUR BABY'S HEAD COULD BE DOWN in your pelvis. You may have a sensation that she's just going to pop out. During the pelvic exam you have around now, your doctor or midwife will assess your progress: how effacement of the cervix is looking, how dilation of your uterus is progressing, and how your baby is positioning, including the station or point of descent in your pelvis.

Are you just sick of the whole thing? The up-at-night, charley-horse-ridden, full-of-someone-else feeling of it all? Have you wondered how you're going to make it another three or four weeks?

Maybe you aren't yet ready for it just to be over, and maybe you won't ever feel that way. There's a lot of paradox for me at this stage of pregnancy. The wonder of having another person inside of me has worn off, replaced by a dull annoyance with the whole situation. I'll have moments of dread, wondering how I will do it once the baby's born and demanding my constant attention. Those will be interspersed with pockets of joy, when I consider how much I don't deserve the blessing of another soul to care for.

As you ride the roller coaster of physical setbacks and emotional contradictions, don't forget to grasp Mary's hand. She's been there, and she's walking with you now. Take your hurdles to her, and ask her to lift you over them.

Walking with Mary: The Crucifixion

Standing at the foot of the Cross, Mary must have experienced the height of paradox. Her son, the baby she had carried and cuddled, had been tortured and was being killed as the worst kind of criminal.

We know Mary was without sin, but frustration and confusion are feelings, not sins. She had to wonder just what in the world God was thinking, just how this would work out for good. Her yes, from the foot of the Cross, is one that speaks to me when I'm feeling most challenged with life.

Mary took a moment of ugliness—the defining moment of humanity's ugliness—and accepted it. She didn't understand it. She didn't like it.

Can I say yes with the same trust in God's will for me? Can I give him the moments of misery and the instants of insanity? Can I let him carry me even though I long to do things myself, on my own, without any help?

One Small Step

As Catholics, we begin and end every prayer with the Sign of the Cross. It's part of our faith tradition. This week, focus on the Sign of the Cross as a prayer in its own right. Trace a cross on your husband's forehead before he leaves for work (if that's too weird, simply do it in your mind), and tell him you are praying for him. For many husbands, seeing the discomfort of their wives at the end of pregnancy (and during labor and delivery) is a version of standing at the foot of the Cross. Ask Mary to remain close to you and your husband as you journey closer to meeting this baby.

Faith Focus

At his Angelus address on September 13, 2009, Pope Benedict XVI said,

> The Virgin Mary, who believed in the word of the Lord, did not lose her faith in God when she saw her Son rejected, abused and crucified. Rather she remained beside Jesus, suffering and praying, until the end. And she saw the radiant dawn of his Resurrection. Let us learn from her to witness to our faith with a life of humble service, ready to personally pay the price of staying faithful to the Gospel of love and truth, certain that nothing we do will be lost.

How ready am I to pay the price of faithful adherence to the gospel? What can I do, right here and right now, to live a life of humble service to those around me?

It's so easy to sneak away from the pain and suffering in front of me. I don't want to watch it; I have enough other things to worry about! What Mary shows me, though, is a better way, a way of sorrow leading to joy.

Mary embodies, once again, the hope of the world. She carried that hope within her for nine months, just as you're carrying your child. She suffered with him. She walked her own painful path to his Resurrection, and she reminds each of us that we too can—and should—persevere.

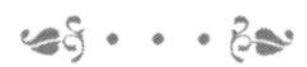

Praying Your Pregnancy

Jesus, it's hard to remember that you have any common ground with a hugely pregnant woman. Help me to feel you by my side and to know that, though you were not pregnant yourself, you surely feel my aches and pains, joys and sorrows, as if they were your own. Amen.

CHAPTER 34

Week 38 (Fetal Age: 36 Weeks)

CONGRATULATIONS! YOU ARE NOW, BY OFFICIAL standards, considered full-term. That is not code for "you should be at max-miserability" or even "let's get this over with," mind you. It's a benchmark of how far you've come. Remember when you first found out about your baby? Does it seem like it was forever ago?

Soon—very soon—you will be holding that baby in your arms. Your journey through pregnancy this time is almost finished.

And yet you might feel like you have so very far to go. Labor and delivery might be looming before you like a bad dream. Whether you've given birth before or not, this time is its own unique experience. It might be similar to your past labors, or it might be completely different.

If you find yourself facing dread countered with longing to have the baby out of you, find comfort in knowing that this is normal and that it will be over and done in a relatively short amount of time, when you step back and view the big picture. In the here and now, it seems impossibly long and drawn out. In a few years (or even as soon as a few months), it will be only a blip in your memory.

Walking with Mary: The Resurrection

Jesus doesn't appear in the Resurrection as a spirit: he comes back as a complete person, body and soul. There's a lesson for each of us in this, especially when we're at a point where we might hate the way our bodies look or feel. The physical has eternal importance. We don't die and leave our bodies behind; they are part of who we are at the most basic and important level.

In the Resurrection, we have a glimpse of Jesus' glorified body. His closest friends don't recognize him until they hear his voice. What does this mean for us, as we look at ourselves in the mirror? To me, it signals that my body is important to God beyond just giving my soul a home for seventy years or so.

Look at your body in wonder: it's housing another human being right now. Look at it with respect: you are made in the image and likeness of God! Your body is not like socks that get worn out and tossed in the trash, but more like your favorite jeans, the ones that grow more comfortable with each wearing.

This week, look to the risen Christ, and see hope in the tangible and touchable. Think of the elation Mary must have felt to see her son again, in a most impossible way. Embrace her hand and ask her for a glimpse of the joy that is to come.

One Small Step

I have always loved how the Catholic Mass is an experience involving all of the senses. There are things to see, of course, and to hear, but also to taste and smell. When you're at Mass this week, pay extra attention to how your senses are engaged.

What do you see as you walk into the church? How does the water in the font feel as you bless yourself? Do you feel God around you? Is there a certain smell to the church itself? What sounds are around you? And how does this sensual imagery—from seeing to hearing to touching to tasting to feeling—change as Mass progresses?

Thank God for the gift of your body, which allows you to experience him in the Eucharist during Mass. Use your body, during Mass, to give God glory in the best way you can, and know that he smiles as he sees you doing it.

Faith Focus

There are days when I struggle to pray "for real." All I can manage is short exclamations, like "Help me," and "Oh Lord, please tell me there's sleep ahead somewhere!"

Except that these are prayers and perhaps some of the most authentic. It is when I'm involving God in my everyday life in the most intimate ways—by calling out to him from the midst of laundry piles and work challenges—that I am really embracing what prayer as conversation really means.

This kind of prayer is called an "aspiration." Pay attention to when you use it, and try to use it more. Rather than shout out a word that sends you to confession or embarrasses you in front of the kids, turn it into a prayer and a plea for help.

• • •

Praying Your Pregnancy

Oh God, this pregnancy is coming to a close, and I'm not sure I'm ready. Just as I was getting myself used to the idea of being pregnant, it's all going to change again. Stand before me in the Resurrection and show me the hope that's always before me. Amen.

CHAPTER 35

Week 39 (Fetal Age: 37 Weeks)

YOUR BABY HAS GROWN SO BIG THAT YOUR UTERUS fills your pelvis and nearly all your abdomen, pushing everything else out of its way. "Uncomfortable" might be too mild a word for the way you're feeling at this point. Are you feeling anxious one minute and excited beyond belief the next? Is it hard to think of anything beyond labor? How is your husband holding up right now?

It's the home stretch, and you're near the end of the first phase of this part of your mothering. Soon you'll be holding her in your arms, wondering what life was like without her.

Don't rush through this time, as tempting as it is to just want it to all be done. Make a memory book or a journal of some kind that you can share with your child when she's older and intensely interested in what you were thinking and feeling right before she was born.

Walking with Mary: The Ascension

Did Mary's heart break just a bit when her son ascended? It marked the end—the real end—of his time on earth, after all, and the last time she would see him here.

Change is exciting, and it's terrifying too. Christ's Ascension marked a change for the early Christians. They had the risen Christ after the horror of the crucifixion. Now he was returning to heaven. What next?

Jesus gives us all a lesson in the Ascension. He goes to where he's supposed to be. Where are we supposed to be? For me, that changes depending on the day or time. Am I supposed to be on the floor with a preschooler reading a book, or am I supposed to be in the kitchen preparing dinner, or at my computer finishing a work project? I can't bilocate (though I keep trying), so I have to choose.

When I look to the Ascension, I see clearly that I'm supposed to be with Jesus. Jesus goes to where he's supposed to be; he doesn't hang around for an extra few years giving his followers extra instructions or backup plans. He's in heaven and I'm not, so it's a little harder to figure it out, but he has given me all sorts of instructions, if only I'll listen. When I open myself to the Holy Spirit and the still, small voice of God, I know the peace of making the right choice.

One Small Step

Turn your eyes to heaven and spend some time with Jesus in the Blessed Sacrament. Find an hour in your week and an adoration chapel in your area, and go and look to heaven. If leaving the house right now is too ambitious, make a special corner, decorated with a pretty cloth, some candles, and some holy objects, and spend some quiet time praying (perhaps starting with the litany in the following section).

Faith Focus

A litany is a prayer that's petition and response, usually with a theme and a repeating response. There are many different litanies. I've included a favorite of mine, which is to the Sacred Heart of Jesus. Responses are in italics, though if you're praying it by yourself, you pray both parts.

Lord, have mercy. *Lord, have mercy.*
Christ, have mercy. *Christ, have mercy.*
God the Father in heaven, *have mercy on us.*

God the Son, redeemer of the world, *have mercy on us*.

(Repeat, "Have mercy on us" after each petition below.)

God the Holy Spirit,

Holy Trinity, one God,

Heart of Jesus, Son of the eternal Father,

Heart of Jesus, formed by the Holy Spirit in the womb of the Virgin Mother,

Heart of Jesus, one with the eternal Word,

Heart of Jesus, infinite in majesty,

Heart of Jesus, holy temple of God,

Heart of Jesus, tabernacle of the Most High,

Heart of Jesus, house of God and gate of heaven,

Heart of Jesus, aflame with love for us,

Heart of Jesus, source of justice and love,

Heart of Jesus, full of goodness and love,

Heart of Jesus, wellspring of all virtue,

Heart of Jesus, worthy of all praise,

Heart of Jesus, king and center of all hearts,

Heart of Jesus, treasure-house of wisdom and knowledge,

Heart of Jesus, in whom there dwells the fullness of God,

Heart of Jesus, in whom the Father is well pleased,

Heart of Jesus, from whose fullness we have all received,

Heart of Jesus, desire of the eternal hills,

Heart of Jesus, patient and full of mercy,

Heart of Jesus, generous to all who turn to you,

Heart of Jesus, fountain of life and holiness,

Heart of Jesus, atonement for our sins,

Heart of Jesus, overwhelmed with insults,

Heart of Jesus, broken for our sins,

Heart of Jesus, obedient even until death,

Heart of Jesus, pierced by a lance,

Heart of Jesus, source of all consolation,

Heart of Jesus, our life and resurrection,

Heart of Jesus, our peace and reconciliation,

Heart of Jesus, victim for our sins,

Heart of Jesus, salvation of all who trust in you,

Heart of Jesus, hope of all who die in you,

Heart of Jesus, delight of the saints,

Lamb of God, who take away the sins of the world, *have mercy on us.*

Lamb of God, who take away the sins of the world, *have mercy on us.*

Lamb of God, who take away the sins of the world, *have mercy on us.*

Jesus, gentle and humble of heart. *Touch our hearts and make them like your own.*

Let us pray:

Father, we rejoice in the gifts of love we have received from the heart of Jesus, your Son. Open our hearts to share his life and continue to bless us with his love. We ask this in the name of Jesus the Lord. Amen.[16]

• • •

Praying Your Pregnancy

Jesus, though you're in heaven, you still care so deeply about all of us on earth. Help me to remember that you love me as though I'm the only one in your life. Guide me closer to your heart so that I may better do your will. Amen.

CHAPTER 36

Week 40 (Fetal Age: 38 Weeks)

THOUGH THIS IS THE LAST CHAPTER IN THIS SECTION, you may not deliver your baby for another week or two. On the other hand, you might have already delivered your baby and are reading this because you feel an obligation to have read it all. (And bless your heart for that.)

It's tempting to start to write about labor, but since there's a whole section about that, I'm going to refrain. I'm going to write, instead, about your husband. Your husband is probably just as excited—maybe more so—to meet your baby at last. After all, you've been uniquely connected to your child for quite a while now, and your husband's been the outsider and observer.

In the next few weeks, Daddy may find it challenging in ways that you don't and ways he can't express. There's an adjustment for all of you, and the best thing you can do, despite your inclination to the contrary, is to remember your marriage.

Look at that man you married, and remember the reasons you fell in love. Think back to what he loved about you in the early days. Those things still exist, but you have both grown and changed—maybe a little, maybe a lot. There's a big bunch of change in front of you as your love sits before you as an entirely new person, and there will be a temptation to put your marriage on the back burner while you attend to this demanding little addition to your family.

Don't do it! Your vocation as wife is first, and your vocation as mother is strengthened by the love you and your husband share. Your relationship with him is primary and feeds those relationships you have with your children.

Walking with Mary: Pentecost

Thanks to the Holy Spirit, Mary had Jesus. Thanks to Jesus, we all have salvation.

It seems simple enough. I can't help but think, though, that Mary, as spouse of the Holy Spirit, must have had a deep relationship with the third person of the Trinity. It's not something we read much about, and it's hard to use it as an example in my own marriage, or even in my own life.

I think it probably involved how she said yes to God so much. There are many times, in my own life, when I could say yes.

"Yes, I'll help you (fill in the blank with whatever I'm not doing) right now."

"Yes, I'll stop what I'm doing and listen to you talk."

"Yes, I'll trust God that he will provide."

Saying yes to the Holy Spirit working in us empowers us to do things more like Jesus did. It opens us to God's grace in our lives. It frees us from having to come up with the decisions to do the important things in life.

Mary knew all this, and she guides us as we struggle with it. Ask her, as you meet the challenge of the end of your pregnancy, to help you accept the Holy Spirit's help.

One Small Step

The Bible is the inspired Word of God, and we do well to spend time with it every day. Saint Jerome even went so far as to say, "Ignorance of Scripture is ignorance of Christ."[17] This week, read the account of Pentecost from the Bible, in Acts 2:1–13. Reflect on it, and make time to journal about it, apply it to you current state of life and experience of pregnancy. Let the Holy Spirit work in you and through you.

Faith Focus

Pope Benedict XVI, in his address to the Roman Curia on Christmas of 2008, shared this: "The Holy Spirit gives us joy. And he is joy. Joy is the gift that sums up all the other gifts. It is the expression of happiness, of being in harmony with ourselves, which can only come from being in harmony with God and with his creation."

Harmony isn't something that I usually feel at the end of pregnancy. In fact, harmony is something I struggle with all the time. The Pope reminds me here that it is from the Holy Spirit, and from the joy he brings me, that I will find true harmony.

It is a gift, one that I can decline. The Holy Spirit won't force it on me, but I'll find myself miserable without it.

How can you find joy today? Where is the Holy Spirit pointing you for greater harmony?

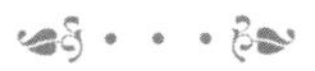

Praying Your Pregnancy

Come, Holy Spirit, come into my life and guide me to the peace you offer. Come, Holy Spirit, and enkindle in me a love that shows itself to others in charity. Come, Holy Spirit, and give me strength to do my duty and embrace the implications of practicing my faith. Amen.

PART TWO

Labor and Birth

ENTIRE BOOKS EXIST TO HELP YOU UNDERSTAND AND approach labor and birth. It is not my intent to try to replace those books with this section. The information I'm including is very general. I'm assuming that if you're the kind of person who's going to read about labor and birth, you already have a book (or ten) that you've read and/or highlighted.

After a brief recap of what you'll likely experience in labor and birth, I'd like to propose a different approach, one that involves our Catholic faith.

Just as we journeyed through the forty weeks of pregnancy, we'll journey through labor and then through birth. Hold out your hand and grab Mary's. Look at a crucifix and unite yourself with the One who really understands pain and discomfort.

After a summary, I'll share a chapter on labor preparation and then one with detailed spiritual practices you can use for your labor experience. For birth, there will also be a summary chapter, and then tips and strategies, followed by spiritual practices. Each chapter will offer my thoughts on preparation and suggest detailed spiritual practices available for your labor and birth experiences.

Let's pause, before we get started, and offer a prayer for guidance and the grace to cooperate with God's will for this time:

Dear Mary, you always said yes, even when it involved pain.
Labor looms ahead of me, and I know it's going to be unlike anything I've ever done before.
Pray for me, Mother of God, that I may follow your yes and turn to your son just as you did.
Guide me toward accepting the graces all around me during this challenging time,
and help me embrace what's ahead despite any fear I may have. Amen.

CHAPTER 37

A Summary of Labor

I HAVE LEARNED, OVER THE YEARS, THAT FEW THINGS can unite a room of women who are complete strangers and turn them into soul sisters like a discussion of labor. I have also observed, though, in part from my own discomfort and hesitation, that this topic is also something I keep quiet about with strangers.

I can't explain the paradox: I'll talk about labor immediately and enthusiastically—how I didn't even realize it was the "real thing" with my first and we barely made it to the hospital—and yet, I hesitate to share with a stranger that I have experienced unmedicated labor three times. Maybe it's that I've heard people go on and on about the joys of epidurals; maybe it's that I can't get over the feeling that, however hard and grueling they might have been at the end, for the most part, my labors have been easy; maybe it's that people have such strong opinions about labor that I hesitate to open myself to criticism.

I have been through labor three times, and though I did it each time without an epidural, I don't think this makes me special or awesome, not by a long stretch! In fact, I suspect that the reason I have only experienced one kind of labor is because my babies have been positioned ideally, for one thing. Epidurals have pros and cons—they're not for everyone, but neither is an all-natural birth. You have to discover, discern, and decide what kind of labor you want and for what reasons.

Labor is an event unlike any other you'll experience. That person inside you—or people, if you're pregnant with multiples—is coming out of you, and it won't be easy, no matter how easy it might sound, or look, or seem later.

Walking with Mary in Labor

When pressed, the first set of mysteries of the Rosary that come to mind to reflect upon when facing labor and delivery are the Sorrowful Mysteries. And yet, I can't help but think of the entirety of the Rosary.

While we have been reflecting for the thirty to forty weeks of your pregnancy on a single set of mysteries of the Rosary, I find myself almost at a loss in this section.

Which mystery should I recommend?

It's impossible to know, without a doubt, how labor will go—how it will turn out, how long it will take, how you will feel at the end, how a million other details will turn out. You just can't tell, for certain.

I'm not someone who takes a lot of comfort from not knowing. The reason I have at least five Google calendars pulled up on my screen as I type this—with a to-do program running along smoothly in the background—is because I like to know for sure, to plan, to be in control. After years of falling flat on my face, I realize I am not the one in control, but it doesn't stop my type-A psycho-organizing mentality from approaching everything from this perspective.

Letting go and letting God is easier said than done. It is at the point when I most need to do this—during labor, for example—when I find the Rosary to be a lifeline of immense proportions. It dangles in front of me, organized into decades and mysteries and prayers that I can slip into like my favorite pair of comfy shoes. It will take me right to Jesus through the best possible avenue, the mother who brought him into this world and knows so well, exactly what I face at the moment when I grasp it in my hands.

Turning to Mary during labor may seem strange to you. I never thought of her actually going through labor until I was in labor with my first child. Did she feel the pains of labor? Was she, at the very least, uncomfortable?

We really don't know. There are theological arguments both ways. I think, though, that it's safe to say, woman to woman, that Mary can walk with us in this journey just as she did through pregnancy. "Without sin" does not mean she was without feeling or without understanding. "Immaculate" does not mean pampered or distant.

Mary is with you as you face this. Are you scared? Are you worried? Are you just unsure? Turn to her. Lean back into her arms. Feel your hand in hers. Trust her to lead you to Jesus and to carry you, if need be, through the hardest parts of what you face during labor and delivery.

Labor: The Short Course

Labor essentially takes place over two to three days. It starts with contractions that move the baby down the birth canal. This first stage of labor is also the longest. It's the stage that had me shaking in my shoes when women would tell me they had been in labor for forty-eight hours.

Your bag of waters may or may not break. You may or may not need to get to the hospital right away. You may or may not be able to get your affairs in order and even calmly entertain yourself for much of this first stage.

In the second stage of labor, you push the baby out. Sounds straightforward, but it isn't always, and it's also far from easy. It was during the second stage of labor that I realized that this baby was coming out of me! Very soon! All of a sudden, motherhood was real in a way it wasn't before, even when I went through it with my second and third children.

With the "prize" so close, I was tempted to give up. I wanted it to stop now! It was during the second stage of labor that my support team was critical. Pushing that baby out took every ounce of mental energy I had, though it was a largely physical experience. Maybe that would make more sense to me if I were more of an athletic person.

I only know about the third stage of labor because of my reference material. According to that, it's the placenta coming out. I do remember this in each of my labors, but it's as a postscript in my mind. In my opinion at the time, the important work, the hard work, was done in stages one and two.

Tools for Labor: Your Support Team

I think there are two essentials for labor, and you need to have them ready before it starts. They are your support team and the right mind-set.

Your first tool for labor is a support team. My husband is always my go-to guy for labor. He knows what I have in mind, what my priorities are, and the areas that cannot be compromised. He also agrees that we need another person, a professional doula, as part of our team—her job is to help him by understanding and explaining, and supporting throughout the labor. Other people I know have their moms or sisters or other women involved in their labors; I have a very strict "only these two people" rule during my labors.

When you determine who's on your support team, you need to discuss your priorities before labor kicks in. Do you care if the whole family shows up to wait in the lobby? Do you feel strongly about medicated versus unmedicated labor? What's important to you when you think about your labor?

Some things you won't be able to control: the time of day, for example. Other things—whether you're having a home birth or a hospital birth, whether you want to have an epidural or not, who you're going to alert that labor's beginning—are worth examining and spending some time thinking about and discussing.

Tools for Labor: Having the Right Mind-Set

I'm not an athletic sort. At the time of this writing, I don't have a regular workout routine, though I have all sorts of signs and signals from my body that I need one, and soon. So comparing labor to an athletic event is a bit unsettling for me, though it is, I think, almost unavoidable. So much of what labor is for your body is comparable to athletics. You're stretching and pushing yourself almost beyond your limits.

There's a prize at the end, too, though it is, arguably, much better than anything you could earn at any athletic event.

In case you don't find yourself inspired by athletic comparisons either, let me offer these words of advice: you must have a positive mind-set.

A friend of mine faces labor strapped to a hospital bed. She's unable to move or get comfortable because of a life-threatening clotting disease she has. This friend has taught me a lot about what it means to embrace your cross. She's also made me realize that how I walk into something like labor—the thoughts I have and the expectations I set for myself—have a lot to do with whether the experience will be positive or negative.

A lot about labor is rough. It's painful. It's . . . well, it's another human being coming out of your body. Enough said!

You can approach it by being scared. You can look at it as something you have to endure to get the prize. You can see it as a step along the road of motherhood.

Or you can see it as an opportunity for grace.

Throughout our lives, there are plenty of things that will arise in front of us and challenge us, especially as they relate to motherhood. Labor isn't the first time you will have an opportunity for grace. You can ignore it. But if you embrace it, if you offer it back to God, what spiritual benefits might you experience?

Only you can answer that. And the answer will be different with each labor.

CHAPTER 38

Preparation for Labor

JUST AS PREPARING FOR A MARATHON OR MAJOR athletic event (or, for that matter, a home renovation) takes many months, so does preparing for labor. It is, in many ways, very similar to a marathon. Your body has to get that baby out, and I'd like to tell you it will be easy and painless. I won't lie. I have no idea how your labor will go . . . and neither do you.

That's the thing with labor—there are no guarantees. That's why it's so helpful to prepare yourself ahead of time, whether you are the sort of person who takes months or if you just happened on this chapter in your last week of pregnancy.

We'll cover three aspects of preparation: mental, physical, and spiritual. I'll also share three preparations that have helped me as I've traveled through labor.

Mental Preparation

It's important for me to understand what's coming. I'm the sort of person who has to plan to be spontaneous, though, so I'm guessing you might be a bit more laid-back.

Knowing what's coming for labor is tricky. Every labor's different, in part because every set of circumstances is different. You are a different person than you were last time, and this baby is a different person than the last baby. If it's your first time through labor, well, you're new to it. You can't possibly know what to expect—the experience of a thing is far different than any reading or observation.

Even with all the unknowns, you can prepare yourself for a few things:

1. Labor is coming. The baby must come out.
2. It won't be easy. It will be hard work.
3. You will have a prize at the end.

I'm not a fan of over-reading about labor, but I do recommend that you find a book that explains the biology of labor in a way that you understand. There are plenty of websites as well.

Know the stages of labor and the possible signs. Speak with your support team, including your doctor, mom friends, doula, or midwife, about any questions you have. Don't rely completely on the answers you find online, and don't let yourself become alarmed.

As a scientifically minded person with a background in agriculture, labor was the most natural thing in the world for me. It was a series of facts and figures and expectations. That said, there is nothing comfortable or comforting about it. Ask my husband: I was not thrilled as the baby was coming out, any of the times I went through it.

There's a comfort in knowing what's possible, in seeing the facts. There's also comfort, though, in knowing that you'll make it through this. This isn't a fatal disease, but a huge athletic event. You'll sweat and work hard, but you'll make it.

Physical Preparation

It might be too late to advise you to believe the books and experts telling you to perform certain stretches and exercises, but if it's not, believe them. Get yourself in shape. Perform your Kegels and squats. Stretch and keep yourself active (but not too active, mind you). I tell you, it will help. It will help a lot.

I also recommend that you consider packing comfort items. There are things that might make labor more comfortable for you, but if they're not with you, they can't help.

During one of my labors, I found myself at the hospital really early in the process. I hadn't brought any reading material or any of my electronics. My husband and I joked that we should have had a PlayStation as we waited for things to get rolling. It was only a few hours, but man, were we bored. Maybe I should advise you to kneel together and pray through that, but I'd be lying if I said that we did that. What I really wanted was a nap, but after all the hookups and interruptions, by the time the medical staff told me I could sleep, I was wide-awake.

Think of what you might want after your labor, too. When it's you and baby in your room, and your husband's gone home to pick up the other kids and/or his deodorant, you might have a devotional, a Rosary, or even just a pair of socks that will make your postpartum time more comfortable. (Or, if you're like me, it will involve a laptop and a camera!)

Spiritual Preparation

Just as you prepare yourself mentally and physically, you need to prepare your soul. Motherhood will take it all out of you over the years. It will demand every ounce of your mental energy, of your physical prowess, and of your faith and hope. Your soul needs to be just as ready as the rest of you.

You can never be completely ready (so don't get worried or obsessive about it). What you can do, first, is to ask for help. Ask your patron saint, Mama Mary, and your guardian angel to help you to be open to the graces God will send to you during labor.

Do you have a special prayer intention, someone or something that's in your heart? Consider offering your labor for this intention. That's a way to give meaning and purpose to your work, and it's also a great gift for whomever you're offering it for.

In the final weeks of your pregnancy, go to confession. Make things right with God, and be open to the graces of your labor. If you are able to attend an extra Mass or two, offer them for a safe delivery and for your own openness to God's will. There will to be hurdles and irritations—maybe even real trials—during your labor. You have a choice in how you respond. Preparing yourself spiritually will arm you for the battle that's coming and get you ready for the buckling down that will have to happen.

Tools for Labor: Prepare Your Space

You may not be going to a medical facility to give birth: you may be staying home. Wherever you labor, you'll need to prepare your space.

This looks different for each of us. I find that I have to prepare my mental space by knowing what's coming and having an idea of the stages and processes of something before it happens.

For your physical space, you may or may not have a lot of control. You may be able to have music playing, but you may not want music. (And you may think you'll want one thing and find the reality is that you want something completely different.) You may want ambiance and low lights, or you may want a high-energy atmosphere while you labor. And it may change at different times of labor.

Your spiritual space is best prepared by quiet prayer. I know this seems like the impossible, but it can be done.

So how do you prepare, when so much is up in the air and subject to how you feel in the moment? Pack or set aside items that speak to you and comfort you. If your favorite statue or crucifix isn't quite appropriate for a trip to the hospital, maybe you can find something that's a bit better and will have the same outcome for you. You may know that a certain piece of clothing—such as a robe or slippers—will be comforting regardless. There may be a pillow or a blanket that will help you feel more at home or comfortable.

Tools for Labor: Prepare Your Spouse (and Yourself)

There is a special challenge for the dads in the crowd. He's about to watch the woman he loves, the woman he would probably die to protect, go through something so rigorous and unimaginable that he'll feel pretty helpless. He might feel like there's nothing he can do to help, and he might not know or have any idea what he can do to comfort you, support you, and help you during your labor.

It's not easy to talk labor with a guy, especially if you have a type-B introverted man in your life. For our second labor, my husband and I had a doula involved. A doula's a labor coach, of sorts, and she told us, up front, that she saw making my husband look good in the delivery room as her primary job.

My husband told me, after our first child was born, that he could barely keep himself from crying as our baby came out. It was such an amazing, life-changing experience for him to see his child born that he was completely unable to do more than hold my hand and stand there.

For our second and third children, having the doula to coach me and my husband really brought us together during the labor experience in a way that still makes us chuckle as we remember those times. Labor became, thanks to the help of someone else, a uniting experience, instead of a time when I was resenting him and he was wondering just what in the world he could do to ease my workload.

As you and your husband talk about your labor, outline your expectations. What are you looking to get out of labor? What are the priorities for your labor experience? Make sure he understands what you're thinking and expecting. Take time to find out if he has any expectations and what they are. I recommend establishing a code phrase or code words that signal, to him and you, that you're willing to give on your priorities.

Women in labor are very susceptible to suggestion. I remember, during my first pregnancy, being told that a woman who maintains that she wants unmedicated labor can be asked, during labor, "Do you want an epidural?" and hear, instead, "You are not doing a good enough job on your own, so you obviously need drugs."

I don't share that example to color your opinion about medicated births, but rather to demonstrate that you need to be prepared—and so does your husband. It's possible you will not be in a rational state of mind during labor. Your body has a lot of work to do, and I think brainpower is used to make that work happen, . . . which is why your support team and your husband are so critical to you!

Tools for Labor: Prepare Your Family

I have a rule with labor: you'll find out when the baby's born. Since we have other children, there are a few family members who end up finding out that we're heading to the hospital, but I've been very strict with my communications to them: do not come to the hospital.

For me, labor is an experience my husband and I share. I know there are very interested parties among the future grandparents and aunts and uncles. I know we have close friends who would love to be supportive. For me, that support takes the form of asking them to pray for me and to know that I need to be lifted up and held close in prayer during the final weeks of pregnancy. I ask them to be open to the Spirit and to pray when I come to mind.

But I make it clear: I don't want them there during labor. That's just for my husband and me.

It's not meant to be insulting, but I know myself well enough to know that I will only get annoyed. Labor is an intense mental exercise, even as it is incredibly (and understandably) physical. I'm not a natural athlete and I hate to sweat. I would much rather play on my computer or read a book than go run a mile or work out.

Spend some time and determine what your priorities are. Do you want your family to be in attendance? Is there a special person besides your husband (and any medical staff) who you'd like to support you in labor and delivery? Does your husband have a strong opinion about it?

It's far better to be prepared—and to have your family clear about your expectations—than it is to have a terrible experience or to insult someone unintentionally when you're in the midst of one of the most important times of your life.

You will want to spend some time with your older children to prepare them for the experience of you going to labor. It's a scary thought that you will be in the hospital, if you're going there; and if they see you in pain, it will be disturbing as well. What can you do to help them feel reassured? How can you prepare them spiritually before labor? Empower them and talk to them so that they feel like participants, instead of feeling helpless and scared in the waiting room or at a relative's home.

CHAPTER 39

Spiritual Practices for Labor

LABOR CAN UNITE US MORE FULLY WITH CHRIST IN various ways. Here are my suggestions. Adapt them, combine them, and use them as they speak to your heart and soul and situation.

The Paschal Mystery

When we refer to the paschal mystery, we're talking about the suffering, death, and Resurrection of Jesus. It's represented in that time between the Last Supper on Holy Thursday and the Resurrection on Easter Sunday.

We are Easter People, it's true, but Easter is only possible because of Good Friday. Consider that as you enter your own passion during labor that Jesus walked this way, too.

There is a lot of pain and suffering during pregnancy and especially labor. You can't complete it without dying to yourself at some level. You die to yourself—to your natural tendencies, to your immediate desires, to your comfort—and experience great pain, and this brings new life into the world!

The world will never be the same after your labor is over. Whatever the outcome, however unexpected parts of it may be, you are making an eternal impact on humanity.

The paschal mystery calls you to contemplation on Jesus's journey to Easter morning. If that seems too distant, put yourself in his mother's shoes, or picture yourself as one of the disciples. Mary was Jesus' first disciple, the person who followed him before he was even born. Her yes brought him to each of us, and it is through her that we can continue to find him, even in the throes of labor.

As you experience your body's laboring, think about Jesus at various stages of his passion. Picture him hanging on the cross. It was only three hours, but to those at the foot of it (and to him, without a doubt), it must have been a long three hours. The time leading up to it—the suffering, the anticipation, the emotions underneath—must have made it feel everlasting.

What must have gone through Mary's mind as she watched her son make the ultimate sacrifice? How was her own sacrifice colored by the suffering she saw in him? Did she grab John's hand and squeeze? Was she able to look away, to ever forget the image of her boy's body tortured and left to die?

Labor is a lot like standing at the foot of the cross, and you can use this time to grow closer to Jesus and Mary. Let them into your suffering. Reach for their hands as you feel excruciating pain and frustration. Grab on to his cloak and let him help you carry this cross. Look to Mary, as you hold your baby, and thank her for her help in leading you closer to her son.

Stations of the Cross

Reflecting on the paschal mystery leads to the Stations of the Cross. Whether you use a set of images, a prayer book, or your imagination, this devotion is appropriate.

You might modify it to fit your circumstances. Maybe your husband will want to pray it with you . . . or maybe you will want to pray it privately, by yourself.

If you have audio capabilities—an mp3 player or computer—you could find free downloadable versions of the Stations, with reflections on each station.

The Rosary

In the Rosary, I find so much to help me contemplate labor. After our discussion of the paschal mystery and the Stations of the Cross, you might think I'm going to push the Sorrowful Mysteries, and those are good. They tie in well with the suffering. However, all the mysteries of the Rosary are so interlinked, so woven together, that I find a contemplation on the Sorrowful Mysteries leads, without fail, to the Glorious Mysteries. From there, I find myself thinking of Mary holding her infant son, and then I'm in the Joyful Mysteries. As he grows, I'm in the Luminous Mysteries.

Using the Rosary—the full twenty decades or one set of mysteries or even one single mystery—during labor gives you something to grip. I think of it as grabbing Mary's hand and holding on tightly. She's been here just as you have—she gave birth. There's tradition stating that she didn't feel pain, but I don't care. In her complete humanity and in the graces she received as the Mother of God, I can't help but believe that she knows. Her prayers are powerful, too, so praying with her during labor surrounds you in a special way with the very best kind of graces.

As we've walked through pregnancy using various mysteries of the Rosary, so it's possible to travel through labor. If it helps you to think of the finish line, pray the Joyful Mysteries and think of holding the baby. If it helps you to unite your suffering and focus on the pain, embrace the Sorrowful Mysteries. Lift yourself with Christ in the Glorious Mysteries. In the Luminous Mysteries, think of your pain as lighting the way, leading you closer to heaven.

Chances are, during the hours you're in labor, you'll have ample time to consider each set of mysteries in various lights. You may find yourself just dryly praying, feeling as though you're merely reciting the words. Don't be tempted to give up. (Wouldn't that be great for the devil if you stopped?) Do the best you can with where you are mentally and spiritually. If all you can manage is to say a Hail Mary or two while clutching something, do that. The number of prayers isn't the heart of the Rosary: contemplation on the life of Christ is.

If you have an mp3 player of some sort, use it. The audio is very soothing and can guide you through the prayer without you having to worry about remembering the words or counting the prayers. I find I'm led along the path of the Rosary, and I am accompanied by Jesus and Mary in my journey through labor. Check out the free downloads available from Rosary Army[18] and fill your mp3 player before you head to the hospital.

Bearing Someone's Special Intention

In my last labor, I had a very special intention in my heart. I offered my labor for this intention. I found, throughout labor, when I was tempted to complain or even mentally bash the whole experience, that I would remember this intention.

There's something powerful—and intimate—about using our suffering and pain to help another (or even ourselves). It is prayer as an experience beyond words. It is, in many ways, a way of drawing closer to God through the unspoken conversation we have with him. God knows our hearts, and he wants more than anything to be united to us.

Labor can be harrowing in many ways, physically and emotionally. Using the focus of a special intention—perhaps one that no one else knows about—can give it a spiritual purpose that might help to take you beyond the present pain and discomfort.

Holy Images

Holy cards are highly transportable and can be very inspiring. There are a variety of other images that come to mind too, including some that are used in various apps I have on my electronic devices. Maybe you'll have a book with a particularly moving image. A small icon that speaks to your heart is also appropriate.

You might use this image or images to take your mind off your suffering or to give your pain a purpose. Labor is grueling and long, and focusing on different parts of a holy image may feed your soul as your body does its work. Our bodies are never separated from our souls, so feeding our soul gives us strength to continue our labor.

Turning to the Saints

There are many saints associated with childbirth, many more associated with pregnancy, and even more who have special patronages associated with suffering. I encourage you to start, though, with a saint you know, whether it's your patron saint or another one you feel particularly drawn to. Use your time in labor to ask for their intercession and to reflect on different parts of their life.

Saints are known for their lives of heroic virtue. They were not perfect, though. I find hope in that—there's hope even for me, and for those I influence and come into contact with!

Put your labor under the patronage of a special saint. If you're not sure whom to choose, or if you want to have a saint "choose you," try an online saint's name generator.[19]

The Word of God

Why not turn to your Bible? The psalms are a great place to start. They cover the wide range of human emotion and experience. There's joy and rage, confusion and pain, euphoria and worship. It's a great snapshot of pregnancy, in many ways, and they would make quite a companion while in labor.

In the gospels, you'll find the account of Jesus's life and ministry. Reading the gospels during labor might give you a focus you wouldn't have had otherwise and might bring Jesus to life through his own words and your experience in labor.

Exploring other parts of the New Testament, such as Paul's letters to the Ephesians or Corinthians, may be helpful, too. Check out the Book of Wisdom and mine through Proverbs and Sirach. Looking for an adventure to get your mind off the adventure in your body right now? Try one of the books of Maccabees or even Acts of the Apostles.

Spiritual Reading

Here I'll mark myself as a bona fide Catholic nerd, because to me, labor equals a chance to dive into some spiritual masterpiece I've been putting off or haven't gotten to. I'm not saying I have actually read a great Catholic masterpiece during labor, but I usually have one with me. Recently, I read *Introduction to the Devout Life* by Francis de Sales and was struck by how relevant it was to me. It was written in the seventeenth century, and yet I felt like Saint Francis was over my shoulder, speaking directly to me, a married woman living in a very different world five centuries after him.

Word by Word

Sometimes, all you can do is cling to a single word. Whatever the prayer or phrase you choose (I tend toward the Hail Mary), spend a breath or two on each word.

CHAPTER 40

Tips and Strategies for Birth

YOU'VE DONE IT!

Now what?

I thought the feeling was isolated to my first child, especially since I had never really had a fondness for babies before nor had I worked with them. I assumed, with my second and subsequent children, that I would have a clue, that this feeling of "now what?" wouldn't surface.

I was wrong.

Each child is his own person. You are a different person than you were (or will be) with any other child.

Enjoy this time. There's so much to cherish—and so much to hate. If you're nursing, or if you find yourself experiencing NICU, or if you face one of a thousand other hurdles, you might have a nagging doubt.

In some books, this time is called the "tenth month." Life with a brand-new infant is far different than life without one, whether or not she's your first.

In many ways, there's no way to prepare. It's an active, busy, and exhausting time. In other ways, having the right mind-set—as with labor—can go a long way toward relieving your stress. Gripping God's hand through it all—the poopy explosions, the aftermath of pain, the recuperation, the sleeplessness—will keep you on track.

You have many adjustments to make with the birth of your new baby. She needs you, but so do the other people in your life. You might feel pulled in a thousand directions, or you may feel peace and harmony. You might, in fact, feel all those things—and many others—all at once.

My goal with this chapter is to share some of the tips and strategies that I've found helpful immediately following the birth of a child. I call them "tools for birth," but they could just as easily be dubbed "tips for sanity" or "keeping yourself from losing all sense of lucidity."

Walking with Mary in Birth

Mary certainly held the newborn Jesus and looked at him with the same overflowing expression of emotion you feel as you look at your new infant. Though the specifics of her circumstances were probably far different than what yours are, she still stands in front of you as your mentor and model.

For one thing, she must be very proud of you. You did it! And whatever you face now—uncertainty, possibly some grief, overwhelming joy—she is your companion.

As I prayed the Joyful Mysteries of the Rosary while I nursed my first child, I found myself realizing just how awkward things must have felt for Mary. She was in a stable, surrounded by straw and hay and different animals. While that was probably less uncomfortable for her than it would be for me, it must have been cold. And then the shepherds showed up, their cheeks probably pink from the exertion and the chill in the air.

With my third child, I found myself thinking about the Luminous Mysteries while I was in the hospital. Jesus is a grown man—his mother must have felt like it happened so quickly. I reflected on how quickly my oldest, who was almost six when my third was born, had seemed to transform overnight into my big girl, a helper of immense proportions. I would see her holding her baby brother and realize she would be a young woman so soon.

As I continue to pray the Rosary, I can't help but identify with Mary more and more, in new and different ways, as the lens of my own motherhood changes. It began with the birth of my children. All of a sudden Mary and I were sisters: I was now a member of the Mom Club! And wow, it was much different than I expected, and I found I needed (and continue to need) all the help I can get.

Each set of mysteries gives me new reasons to pause, to look at Mary with renewed respect and awe. Every prayer I send her way ends up changing me a little more and, I hope, making me more and more a woman after her heart.

Don't give up on Mary. Don't turn away from her, or think she doesn't love you, or doesn't long to take you, as often as you want, to her son. Don't think she isn't there every moment of every difficult day.

Share your triumph, your sorrow, and your joy. Grasp the Rosary and let it guide you closer to Jesus's mother, and your mother.

Tools for Birth: Your Support Team

You had a support team for labor, and you need one for birth, too. It may be a similar group of people, and your husband is surely first on the list. As your partner in this parenting adventure, he will be by your side for a good long time—until this little bundle is moving on to her own vocation in life and beyond.

Other members of your support team may include close family members, close friends, or even members of your church. At our parish, we have a ministry where we alert a group of volunteers when we hear about a new baby being born. Those people then contact the family and arrange to show up with a meal at some point.

Consider who your support team is. You'll need physical help in the first few weeks, and that's critical. But after the pain subsides and you're able to move around better, you'll still need to know you have a cushion of people to call on.

Few things can bring a completely rational woman to her emotional knees the way an infant can. (I speak from experience.) You need people you can call and whom you trust. If one of the people on your support team notices that you need a break—or a nap—you need to believe that person. You also need to have a few people you can call and vent to or invite over to hold the baby so you can get a shower (or a nap).

Tools for Birth: Asking for—and Accepting—Help

On my thirtieth birthday, as I was carrying my two-year-old down our farmhouse's steep stairs, I slipped and broke my arm. The following few weeks, I found myself having to accept help with everything from bathing my daughter to preparing meals. I discovered, much to my chagrin, that asking for help is far easier than accepting help.

Why do I fight being the person on the receiving end of others' generosity and their ministering? Maybe it's human nature . . . or mom nature, because I find that I fight it when I'm postpartum too. In many ways, I'm not so different from the three-year-old who insists, despite all evidence to the contrary, that she can do it herself, with escalating voice and acrobatic theatrics.

For me, asking for help is hard, and accepting it is even harder. What I need to remember, though, is that it is a great blessing to allow others to minister to us. If you've ever gone above and beyond in helping someone else—or if you've ever done something seemingly small and inconsequential only to be thanked as though you've gone above and beyond—then you know the blessing. It's embarrassing sometimes. It's nice, though, to be the person helping.

I try and remind myself of that when I answer the phone and someone asks if I need a meal. I try and bite back the "no, thanks, we're fine," for the misleading half-truth it is. We might be fine—we have food somewhere in the house, after all—and we might be thankful, but I'm doing a disservice to the person offering and perhaps even to my family, who might just be ready for a dinner other than cereal and SpaghettiOs® and frozen casserole surprise.

After I have a baby, one of my sisters-in-law makes a point of stopping over to pick up all my laundry. It was a bit disconcerting the first time she did it, but I've learned not to argue with her. She brings it back, smelling fresh and folded so nicely, and often someone else shows up to put the full baskets of clothes away.

Family members are harder to say no to (at least in my experience), but if you aren't fortunate enough to have family close by, consider the help of your parish family or circle of friends as something integral and needed. You might have to ask, and I know that's hard. You definitely have to be able to say yes to the help that's offered, however tentatively.

Tools for Birth: Sleep

In college, I had a motto: "There'll be plenty of time for sleep when I'm dead." Twenty-odd years, a husband, and three kids later, I look back at the person who actually believed that and laugh.

I've always operated well with less sleep than the people around me. The first two weeks after my first child was born, I probably averaged three or four hours of sleep per night. And then, because the regime didn't let up, I crashed. Hard.

I started to realize the importance of sleep somewhere between my first and second children. I noticed my health was better, my attitude was better, my life was better . . . and my outlook hinged on having enough sleep and being rested.

With an infant, this is nearly impossible. I know, oh how I know. As I write this, I have a nine-month-old who's not sleeping through the night—he sleeps in stretches of four hours quite often, but I'm still getting up in the middle of the night. I've been sleep deprived for quite a while, because at least once or twice a week, I forget to have the three-year-old go potty before tucking her in, and I'm up with her in addition to being up with the baby.

I've learned to let go of some things in order to carve out time to sleep. I'm not usually able to nap during the day, but when it's bad enough and the room is dark enough, I can.

In the first few months of a baby's life, sleep is essential . . . for you. The baby may or may not follow what all the "experts" say about sleep patterns, but you need to make sure you are getting enough sleep so that you can function. If that means you ask for help, do it . . . and then accept the help that's offered. If it means you wait to do laundry, even though it's so much easier to do it while the baby naps, then wait, and take a nap yourself. One of the most used pieces of advice every new mom hears is to nap when the baby naps. I've had varying levels of success with this, postpartum being one of the only times in my life when I've been willing to shut my eyes during daylight hours.

Life doesn't look right when you don't have enough sleep. I'm not suggesting that you will have enough sleep before your child's eighteen, but don't let that be your fault or because you have not taken advantage of the time you have. Especially if you notice, as I do, that the likelihood of depression or irrational behavior increases exponentially when you're sleep deprived, make sure you come up with ways to get some sleep!

Tools for Birth: Prioritize

You have to take care of certain things, regardless of how you feel. The baby's needs have to be met, and so do yours. The rest of your family needs certain things from you. Oh, and there's something crunchy all over the floor, the laundry's piling up to the ceiling, and the dishes can't wash themselves.

In the first weeks of your baby's life, your priorities will be different—and need to be different—than they are normally. This is your "new normal," and it's a transitional time. Be clear with yourself—and your family—that it won't last forever and that it's okay that housework or other work that usually gets done isn't going to get done with the same frequency.

What's most important? What can others help with? What can wait?

There's nothing like a new person living in the house to throw all your former routines and priorities up in the air. Things have changed without a doubt, and they will continue shifting for the rest of your life. You are tied to this baby in a whole new way, and your ways of doing business have to reflect that.

When I'm feeling most overwhelmed, I find that spending quiet time in prayer (preferably before the Blessed Sacrament) with a notebook is the best way to start thinking out my prioritization challenges. If it's easier to approach things from a goal-setting standpoint, do that. Use a calendar, or just dust off a blank notebook and make good old-fashioned lists of three goals per day. (Even that might be a bit ambitious, come to think of it.)

I try to limit myself to three things per day even when I'm not freshly postpartum. Granted, I have them categorized, such as home, errands, phone calls, and sometimes a column for work, but I have learned over years of flirting with burnout that my to-do list has to be achievable. What's achievable on any given day or in any given season of motherhood takes discernment and thought.

Your top priority should be to God in prayer, though it does not have to be a quiet time where you sit down and do nothing else. (That might seem ideal, but it probably also feels impossible right now.) Find a way to turn a repetitive task—changing a diaper, walking to the sink, brushing your teeth—into a prayer. When one of our children was an infant, I got into the habit of saying a Hail Mary every time I went up or down our stairs. Though we have since moved into a one-story house, I still catch myself praying a Hail Mary when I'm going up or down stairs.

Prioritizing could be the subject of an entire book, and it warrants your fullest attention. Keeping in mind that your priorities will change and knowing what your priorities right now are will guide you as you set goals and work toward following God's plan for your life.

Enjoying Baby

Admittedly, I'm not a baby person. I have an arsenal of responses for anyone who offers to let me hold their infant. With my own babies, though, I am always shocked (and delighted) that I seem to suddenly be a baby person. They like me! I like them back!

Oh, and did I mention I hate them? I'd feel guilty if I didn't admit that publicly. Newborns are a love-hate situation for me. I love nursing and feeling their small weight against me, but I hate the never-ending demands and the loss of brainpower that inevitably results from dealing with a small person who's more narcissistic than me. It's not that the newborn can help it, I know, but it's more a reminder of my many flaws as a person.

Part of what I most enjoy about one of my new babies is how much I see that I've grown—and how much more I know I will grow. They stretch me to reach higher and harder for God's hand and to lean farther and faster into his arms. God truly carries me through the postpartum time, and he has an army of assistants, from my guardian angel to my patron saints to my friends and family.

CHAPTER 41

Spiritual Practices for Birth

I COULD NOT SURVIVE MY POSTPARTUM TIME without God. Period.

That said, I probably take his name in vain more during this period than any other. . . . There's something about that certain note a wailing newborn can reach—for no apparent reason—that just puts me over the edge. The combination of a demanding infant and clueless (or so they seem to me) family is usually enough to drive me to God with my fists thrashing and the words flowing from my lips in an angry stream.

My prayer for you is that you reach for him and rest in his arms. Unload your cares on him: he's far better suited to carrying your burden than anyone else.

These spiritual practices may or may not speak to you. Adapt them as needed, and combine them as you're inspired to do so. Know that you will be in my prayers in a special way through this difficult and joy-filled time in your mothering.

Holding Mary's Hand through the Rosary

In the Rosary, I am called beyond myself, past the present strife to the eternal. Whether it's a screaming baby or an impossible deadline, it is in the Rosary, however imperfectly prayed, that I find myself grabbing Mary's hand and looking in her eyes.

I struggle with seeing Mary on a pedestal. If she's so perfect, what can she have in common with me? If she's so blessed and graced, how can she stoop down to spend any time with someone as sinful and selfish as I am? If she's such a yes woman, how can she possibly understand my tendency to say no?

There's room to keep distance from Mary, because I am earthy and she is flawless. She seems so perfect on her pedestal: why would she want to help me with my mundane problems? There's a temptation to see my puke-covered, unshowered, and disheveled self as completely different from her.

Nothing could be further from the truth.

Mary was completely human. She felt frustrated and angry and overwhelmed, to be sure. The difference between us is that she chose not to sin and give in to the temptations underlying the challenges of motherhood. She can inspire me, if I let her get close enough to be real. She can lead me closer to her son and her spouse, the Holy Spirit, if I open my hand to hers.

The Rosary gives me a starting place for a relationship with Mary. As I meditate on the mysteries of her son's life, I find myself looking for her and wondering about her response to various parts of her life. Sometimes I think about what she would do in my place.

When I'm moving Rosary beads through my hands or counting on fingers as I'm up to my ears in some project, I think about Mary looking over my shoulder. I picture her smiling and encouraging me. She and I have common ground in her son, though he's often not the first one I think about. Jesus, as Mary's son, becomes more interesting to me as I continue my own journey of motherhood. What kind of child was he? Was he as daring and unencumbered as my own son is? Did he appreciate the beauty of the weeds on the side of the path? Did he run and scream and thrive?

There is so much in my life as a mother to distract me. There are the millions of things that need to be done and the thousands of things I have to remember. I guess, then, that it's not surprising that I often lose my place as I'm praying, unless I'm using an app or an audio Rosary to help me. It's important to remember that the form is not as important as the intention. God sees you trying and blesses you for it. Mary is cheering you on, pulling you always closer to her son.

Starting Every Day with a Morning Offering

It's a sentence or two, but it can make a difference in my day like few other things. There are times when it's the only formal prayer I'll manage to say in a day. Here's one that I copied from a favorite prayer app:

> O Jesus, through the Immaculate Heart of Mary, I offer you my prayers, works, joys, and sufferings of this day in union with the holy sacrifice of the Mass throughout the world. I offer them for all the intentions of your sacred heart: the salvation of souls, reparation for sin, and the reunion of all Christians. I offer them for the intentions of our bishops and of all the apostles of prayer, and in particular for those recommended by our Holy Father this month.[20]

Consider writing it down and putting it over your kitchen sink, by your toilet, or on your refrigerator so that every time you're there, you remember to pray it. Pray it slowly or quickly, knowing that your prayers are heard by the God who loves you. Maybe you'll want to find different versions and hang them in different parts of your home, so that they'll catch your eye and your attention in different ways on the challenging journey through your day.

Going to the Divine Office

The Liturgy of the Hours (also called the Divine Office) is the official prayer of the Church. By praying throughout the day, you join your prayers with that of everyone else, including the clergy and religious who are required to pray them and the many others who choose to. It is a way of praying constantly. The Liturgy of the Hours uses the psalms, readings from the Church Fathers (the first generation of Christians following the apostles) and spiritual masters, and prayers. (CCC, 1174–1177)

The Liturgy of the Hours has never been easier to pray than it is now that we have modern technology. If you have a mobile device, you can download a variety of apps (iBreviary and Divine Office are my favorites), or you can find the text online. If you have a hard copy of the books, you can use them too. In addition, there are other resources that tap into the Liturgy of the Hours by modifying it slightly, such as what is done by the monthly *Magnificat* magazines (it's also available as an app and online).

The beauty of praying the Liturgy of the Hours is manyfold. You are uniting your prayers with those of the universal church. It's all written down and it's scriptural, so God has room to use his Word to touch you.

Middle-of-the-Night Prayers as a Chance to Bless Someone Else

My second child was having a particularly bad spell with breathing at night, and it was during one of the middle-of-the-night vigils with her that I recalled something someone had recently mentioned about the souls in purgatory needing prayers. As I stumbled out of bed, I felt a strong call to pray for those souls. I punctuated my middle-of-the-night rocking with prayers and found that, though I was still exhausted, I had put my time to another use. Not only was I caring for my child, but I was helping, in some small way, those souls in purgatory.

Sometimes, my middle-of-the-night prayers have no words, because I'm too exhausted to think of them. If I have a special intention, I'll often say a little prayer as I go to bed, committing any of my prayers that night for the intention of my heart.

There's solace, for me, in these still, quiet prayers. Even as my head pounds and my eyes droop, my soul works, and my suffering stands as a blessing for someone else. I find, too, that I am irrevocably changed by this mentality and have a lower tendency to see the interruptions to my sleep as inconveniences when I can view them through the lens of an eternal blessing for someone else.

A Novena of Hours

Novenas are typically prayers that are repeated each day for nine consecutive days. I have no shame in adapting things though, and have experimented with other forms of nine. Nine minutes, nine hours, nine weeks, nine months . . . they all offer an opportunity for focusing and refocusing on turning to God with our needs and intentions.

During this new-infant phase, there are plenty of hazy times with hours that stretch before you. Take nine of them and pray a simple pattern of an Our Father, a Hail Mary, and a Glory Be at the top of each hour. See how it strengthens you for the battle of that stretch of time.

PART THREE

Baptism

FOR ME, FEW THINGS EXPRESS THE JUBILATION AND excitement of a new baby the way a Baptism does. In our small parish, we can schedule Baptisms during Mass. During the Our Father, our priest takes the baby up to the altar.

During that Mass, when my baby becomes one with the Body of Christ and the Church, I usually battle tears. There's my child, coming home. There's my Church family, welcoming him. Surely Baptisms must be one of God's favorite things.

The first Christians were baptized as adults and brought their children in later to be baptized, promising to raise them to follow Christ. It's a tradition that continues to the present day.

I almost didn't hold a reception after our third baby's Baptism. It was a Saturday in December and half the family couldn't attend because of weather and other obligations. My husband gently reminded me, though, that planning the Baptism reception is just about the only kind of event I enjoy planning. He also reminded me, mostly with his eyes, that this was a once-in-a-lifetime event.

We are only born into the family of God once. It's worth celebrating, commemorating, and remembering.

It's also worth acknowledging with at least as much preparation and thought as the rest of your baby's early life. You had to get him into this world, but you want to get him into the next world, too!

In this section, you'll find a brief overview of Baptism, including an examination of what the Catholic Church teaches about this sacrament. Then we'll talk preparation—which can begin before your baby's even born—and we'll conclude with a chapter of reflection related to Baptism.

Walking with Mary to Baptism and Beyond

Your child's Baptism is a cause to party, to celebrate, to rejoice! It is also a time to turn to Mary as never before.

When her own son was baptized, it marked the beginning of his mission, his going away from her. There must have been pride swelling in her heart even as the pang of seeing him leave struck her.

Your child is in your care now. She depends on you for everything, but that will soon change. You are making a solemn pledge during her Baptism, and it can seem like an overwhelming responsibility.

Getting your family to heaven—the call we all seek to answer in our vocations as wives and mothers—is a big order. Who better to turn to than Mary? For one thing, she's already in heaven. For another thing, she's right beside us.

Yes, I realize that is a contradiction, but isn't it a lovely contradiction? Isn't it wonderful to imagine that the woman on Satan's most-hated list is protecting each of us? Don't you just beam when you picture the party Mary must host in heaven?

It's irresistible to turn to the heavenly host during something big like Baptism. It's logical, in fact. But let's not forget to keep Mary by our side through the small steps that take us to the next big milestones. Before your child's First Communion, you have many years of harrowing parenting ahead of you. Before your child's Confirmation, you have hours of debates and praying. Before any other sacraments or graduations, you have miles and miles to go.

Mary is there, leading you ever closer to her son. She's there with you, every Hail Mary you breathe, every mystery you contemplate. She will surely carry your prayers to heaven and help you cooperate with all the graces you need to be the mother God has called you to be.

CHAPTER 42

Overview of Baptism

OUR PRIEST ALWAYS JOKES THAT WE NEED INFANT Baptism to rid the world of pagan babies. This never fails to make parishioners smile, though it does muddy the waters a bit.

Where does the practice of infant Baptism come from? Is it really necessary?

The short answer is that it's only as necessary as you're willing to take responsibility. Your newborn can't speak for herself yet. Your role during Baptism, then, is to promise to raise her in such a way that she will grow into the baptismal vows.

What the Church Teaches about Baptism

The Catechism of the Catholic Church explains Baptism this way:

> Holy Baptism is the basis of the whole Christian life, the gateway to life in the Spirit (*vitae spiritualis ianua*), and the door which gives access to the other sacraments. Through Baptism we are freed from sin and reborn as sons of God; we become members of Christ, are incorporated into the Church and made sharers in her mission: "Baptism is the sacrament of regeneration through water in the word." (*CCC*, 1213)

The *Catechism* also addresses infant Baptism, in paragraph 1231:

> Where infant Baptism has become the form in which this sacrament is usually celebrated, it has become a

> single act encapsulating the preparatory stages of Christian initiation in a very abridged way. By its very nature infant Baptism requires a post-Baptismal catechumenate. Not only is there a need for instruction after Baptism, but also for the necessary flowering of Baptismal grace in personal growth. The catechism has its proper place here. (*CCC*, 1231)

Infant Baptism, then, is perfectly acceptable. In most of the Catholic circles I've been in, it's the norm. I was not raised Catholic, though, and the question of infant Baptism raises issues. Wouldn't it be better to wait until the children are old enough to decide for themselves? In the paraphrasing of my mother-in-law, "No. They might decide not to!"

I once read the story of a woman's conversion to the Catholic Church. She had been an active atheist. In the course of studying Church teachings and learning about the Catholic faith through RCIA classes, she realized she had been baptized in a Catholic Church.

She hadn't been raised Catholic. She was, in fact, raised with nothing, no faith of any kind. She called herself atheist and spent much of her young adulthood mocking and ridiculing Christians.

The power of Baptism, though, the indelible mark on her soul (*CCC*, 1317), could be a large part of what brought her back to Christianity.

Who knows? Only God.

As parents, we want to give our children the very best. It follows, then, that as Catholic parents, we want to prepare them for the next life, even as they are beginning to live this life. Baptism is a rite of initiation and our calling to be Christ's body in the world.

CHAPTER 43

Preparation for Baptism

THERE ARE A LOT OF THINGS I WOULD LIKE TO change about my life. I have regrets, and there are things that I wish I had thought of as I've parented my children.

One thing that I especially would change is my preparation for my children's Baptisms.

When I was baptized and confirmed into the Catholic Church, I prepared for many months prior, attending classes with our parish priest. Many people prayed for me. I was covered in graces, even though I'll be the first to admit that I had an attitude slightly smaller than a dump truck and a resistance to authority, acceptance, and participation.

I look at myself and see the powers of the sacrament at work. Ten years ago, I was newly baptized. I was a very different person interiorly, and the positive changes that have happened have been possible because of the graces conferred by Baptism and the other sacraments.

As you prepare for your baby's Baptism, there will be plenty of details to juggle. You might be the kind of person who hosts a huge party and celebrates long into the night. You could be cooperating with family traditions or setting new ones.

You are taking on a special responsibility as you bring your child to the church to be baptized as an infant. You are vowing that you'll aid and guide him in his Catholicism. You are giving him to the entire Church family and indicating that you'll accept their help as you shoulder the duties related to raising your child in the faith.

Tools for Baptism: Learn

Learning about your faith—specifically your Catholic faith—is an ongoing process. If you haven't started, I suggest you start now. It's never too late. Pick up a book, or start following some faithful Catholic websites, such as New Advent (www.newadvent.org), the Holy See (www.vatican.va), or the United States Conference of Catholic Bishops (www.usccb.org). Your parish may have a website with links to other local and relevant sites, and you are always welcome to stop by my website (www.snoringscholar.com). Among my favorite Catholic sites are Conversion Diary (www.conversiondiary.com), CatholicMom.com (www.catholicmom.com), the Catholic Portal at Patheos (www.patheos.com/Catholic), and Star Quest Production Network (SQPN) (sqpn.com). Read Catholic periodicals, such as the *National Catholic Register* (www.ncregister.com), *Catholic Lane* (catholiclane.com), *Catholic Exchange* (catholicexchange.com), and your diocesan publications. Consider attending a parish Bible study or even the RCIA classes, where the faith is introduced to those who wish to be confirmed into the Church as adults.

How does this prepare you for your baby's Baptism? First, by making a commitment to lifelong faith learning, you will impact him. You won't be able to help it. What you're reading, experiencing, and thinking about will be part of who you are and what you discuss. Though your baby isn't ready for that yet, the sooner you start beginning the journey of understanding the faith, the more prepared you will be when he begins asking questions.

Tools for Baptism: Pray

Unceasing prayer is easier said than done, though it can become a habit. I once heard a couple mention that their priest advised them to move their toothbrush to a different place than what they were used to and then, when they were looking for their toothbrush to brush their teeth, to get in the habit of saying a prayer, even something as short and easy as, "Hey,

God, thanks for today. Would you mind helping me out with the diaper situation? Help me know and accept your will. See ya. Amen."

Prayer as a habit is critical to your role as your children's first catechist. A catechist is far more than just a religion teacher, though that's often what we boil it down to. The word catechesis comes from the Greek word meaning "echo." It's being Catholic in your very being, in the essence of who you are. It's teaching by doing, by being, and by remembering that you represent Christ to this certain someone, your child. It's the work of the entire Church, not just those who are formally given the job, but it's primarily the work of parents in a very special, God-given way.

In other words, our lives can be—and should be—an echo of our Catholic faith, of who we are and who Jesus calls us to be. We are passing on our Catholic faith, instructing our children, and forming those who come our way, whether they are family members or complete strangers. I've found that catechesis can be summarized as relying on the authority of the Church and attaching our own experiences. Though it involves taking in information, it is just as critical to consider how we spread the Gospel in what we do, how we live, and who we are.

I can't think about this too much, because it makes me want to crawl into the corner and curl up into the fetal position. The task is so huge and I am so small! I'm terrified, stressed, and overwhelmed, all at once. Who am I to have such a critical role in something as important as building someone else's faith? That answer's easy: I'm the parent, and God has designed things so that I am their first teacher. My children will be exposed to Catholicism through the lens of the catechesis my husband and I provide.

From my years of teaching religious education through our parish before I was married and had kids, I know that a plan is only a starting point. There were many times I would walk into the third-grade classroom with a firm outline of how our time together would go. The Holy Spirit, however, would have different ideas.

In my work since then, including working with Confirmation candidates, I've found that the deeper my prayer life, the stronger my connection to the small nudges and the quiet voice of the Holy Spirit. And when the Holy Spirit is at work, stand back. It's going to get good!

Your prayer life may be on the rocks. You may have no idea what to do or how to do it. Start simply and stick with it. Consider using this time prior to your baby's Baptism as a time to start anew in prayer, with vigor and commitment.

Tools for Baptism: Accept and Reflect

Jesus knocks plenty, but I don't always answer. In fact, there's been more than one time when I'm pretty sure, looking back, that I've slammed the door in his face.

I don't know why he keeps coming back.

The graces of the sacraments are more than we can fully understand or appreciate. Don't underestimate your need for them, and don't ignore their ability to bathe your life in grace.

My priest once explained grace to me this way: "So many times, we picture it as being water, poured into a cup," he said. "But it is actually more like the air we breathe, unable to be contained and limited."

I think the reason so many people have their babies baptized and then disappear from Church life until First Communion is that they have no idea of the enormity of what they've just signed up to do. I also think there's a bit of a grace in that: if they didn't have their babies baptized, how many graces would they—and their children—not have? Would they miss a chance later on, as a result of not having been baptized now?

Imagine your child's Baptism as a strong cord tied around his waist. He'll walk around—and perhaps away from the Church. The strength of that cord, though, never diminishes, and it may just be responsible for bringing him back when he goes seeking far away from where you'd like him to be.

Spend some time reflecting before your baby's Baptism. I'm including some questions below, for you to consider as you prepare for this sacrament. Keep a journal and, in addition to the answers you may have for these questions, include your own ideas and notes.

- What memories do you have of your own Baptism? If you were baptized as an infant, what stories were you told about it? What pictures survive, and what do they say to you?
- What importance has Baptism had on your life? On your husband's life? On other loved ones' lives?
- What part did your family play in your faith formation?
- What hopes and dreams do you have for your child?

Godparents

Some families have a bit of a tradition with godparents, and some have views and opinions about what godparents are (or are not) and what their role includes above and beyond what the Church advises.

In the booklet we received when our first child was baptized, *Together at Baptism*, by Robert M. Hamma, there is a clear explanation of what's expected from a godparent, in the eyes of the Church. "The role of godparents is to help their godchild lead a Christian life," writes Hamma, and this should be at the heart of your decision process. Who will inspire your child to live a life with Christianity at the heart of it?

The technical qualifications for the godparents include:

- Being at least sixteen years old
- Being a member in good standing of the Catholic Church (in our parish office we refer to this as a "practicing Catholic")
- Having received Baptism, Confirmation, and the Eucharist
- Not being a parent of the child being baptized.[21]

Often, people choose two godparents, though only one is required, and you can have up to three (though only two will be recorded in the sacramental records the parish keeps). You must have one godparent who meets the qualifications above;

any other non-Catholic Christians selected are referred to as "Christian witnesses."

For one of our children, choosing godparents was easy, natural, and almost automatic. For the others, though, my husband and I had long discussions that spanned months. We consider godparents an extension of our family, even if they are already family. By entrusting our child to other people, we are giving them a gift, even as they give our child the gift of taking on that role.

A few years ago, when I sponsored a friend who was coming into the Church at the Easter Vigil, I received a book about being a sponsor called *Guide for Sponsors* by Ron Lewinski. Though the book is for those who are sponsoring adults coming into the Church, I found that the description of what it means to be a sponsor was just what I had in mind for my children's godparents.

I have modified the statements from Lewinski's book to reflect godparents:

- Godparents represent the Catholic community. As your child grows, godparents are people close by who are living a Christian life, and providing another example of what that looks like and what it means.
- Godparents are companions. In the best scenario, godparents are the trusted adults your child will turn to when she needs to talk or needs advice. Though it doesn't always work that way, we're looking at the ideal.
- Godparents are mentors. Living a life of faith is ongoing. It never ends. There will always be struggles. That's why it's so critically important to have a cushion of people your child will be able to turn to, look to, and hold up as an example of Christian living.[22]

CHAPTER 44

Reflecting on Your Child's Baptism

AFTER YOUR CHILD'S BAPTISM, YOU MIGHT, LIKE ME, have a resounding thought, "Is it really over that quickly?" Pretty amazing, isn't it? One minute, your baby's unbaptized and the next . . . baptized, a Child of God, part of the Body of Christ.

A struggle we face from the parish office is keeping parents and families involved between the big sacraments, beginning with the gap between Baptism and First Communion. As I've found myself squarely within that time period with my own children, I see the challenges from a different perspective.

It's challenging to be involved in parish life when you have young children, whether you're on your first or your fifth. You probably won't become involved with religious education programs until they're older, and with early bedtimes, evening activities are nearly impossible.

Tools for Passing on the Faith: Pray Together

You teach your child about God all the time, though, and you can incorporate prayer at the important junctures of your life (yes, even when they're little), such as waking, meals, and bedtime. We will often pray the Guardian Angel prayer before a long drive, and I try to pray a Hail Mary out loud whenever we hear an ambulance.

Prayer doesn't have to be awkward or stilted or formal. Learn about the different kinds of prayer and incorporate them into your family life. Turn to God in conversation, and as you become more comfortable with this, you'll find that you naturally share it with your child.

Tools for Passing on the Faith: Mass Attendance

Passing on your faith doesn't have to be isolated to activities that involve your parish. Weekly Mass attendance is a must for you, of course. Your small children don't have an obligation to attend until later, but I encourage you to try your best to involve them. I know there are circumstances that make bringing small kids to Mass a unique torture for parents, but it's worth it. Their souls receive graces from the Mass, and you send an important message to your children about priorities when you bring them regularly.

Tools for Passing on the Faith: Sacramental Strength

Nothing prepared me for parenthood as much as becoming a parent. There are a lot of ways to grow stronger as a parent, but none is as important as your own spiritual health. Stay strong in the sacraments by frequenting them often, with regularity. Go to confession as often as you can (even if you haven't committed a mortal sin), and seat yourself in the pew at Mass whenever you can. Sit before the Blessed Sacrament in adoration.

You can't do this alone, or even with your spouse. You need God. He's there, waiting for you, and he's given you the sacraments. Stay strong in them.

Constant Care

During the rite of Baptism, the priest or deacon addressed you and your baby's godparents: "On your part, you must make it your constant care to bring them up in the practice of faith. See that the divine life which God gives them is kept safe from the poison of sin, to grow always stronger in their hearts."[23]

How would you like to help your baby grow in faith? What are the most important elements of your Catholic faith to you?

Conclusion

THIS JOURNEY BEGAN WITH THE SMALLEST—AND largest—of miracles, that of a new human life. As your baby changed, so have you, in ways you may not fully appreciate until you look back on yourself years from now.

From beginning to end, we have had Mary walking beside us. It's an image I carry with me even when I am not pregnant. I find it comforting and less isolating than trying to do it all by myself.

It is my prayer for you and your family that you continue to welcome Mary into your walk through life. You face many journeys ahead of you. There will be, without doubt, pain and sorrow. You are sure to face joy and elation. And then there's the rest of the time: the mundane and boring, the routine and the regular, the ordinary that can bog you down into lukewarmness.

Do not let the lack of a mountaintop fool you into complacency. Do not let the feeling that your journey is tedious tempt you into ignoring the great spiritual challenges ahead of you. Do not fail to turn to God in every moment.

It is not easy, this life we live. It is not meant to be easy. In the challenges, we find ourselves with opportunities to grow closer to our maker, but those opportunities are also found woven into the fabric of our everyday lives. You can find God in the spaghetti dried in your preschooler's hair, in the crazy outfit your kindergartner wears, and in the heavenly off-key trumpet playing of your gradeschooler. Your teen can shed light on deep theological concepts with his constant questioning, and your adult child can teach you how to grow your spirituality.

There will be many, many times when you are tempted—or when you just drift—into a state of non-excitement. That is, I think, Satan's greatest achievement. We forego our silence and our peace for media and tasks and, in that, we lose our sense of the sacred.

Open yourself to the promptings of the Holy Spirit, continue to grow in your faith, and, above all, keep a firm hold on Mary's hand! As you close the covers of this book and continue down the road of parenthood, may Mary continue to be a shining influence on you. Let's close with a prayer for Mary's ongoing intercession.

Mother Mary, stay with me through this journey of parenthood. Help me to turn to your son with every challenge that comes my way. Guide me in the path to accepting God's will for my life and for this child. Pray for me, Mary, and hold me throughout the days and years ahead. Amen.

Afterword

I DON'T USUALLY PAY MUCH ATTENTION TO TABLOID obsessions with movie stars' procreative activities. How seriously can we take reports that Joan Rivers has birthed an alien baby, after all? A recent news story about Katie Holmes caught my eye, though, because I thought popular reaction to her potential pregnancy was a telling sample of modern women's ambivalence toward motherhood.

Holmes was rumored to have said that she would love to give her daughter the gift of a brother or sister. Many popular bloggers, however, exploded with outrage at the very idea of becoming pregnant for this reason. Pregnancy is an enormous burden, they explained, not to be taken on lightly, and certainly not to be taken on for the good of our existing children.

In popular opinion, it appears, the "important issues" to consider before becoming pregnant are the changes to your body, the burden of breastfeeding, getting up at night, paying for diapers, shoes, and college, and the emotional toll of raising a child to adulthood. In the end, it looks like a simple cost analysis, in which the parents do the giving and the kids do the taking.

When we consider pregnancy and motherhood this way, it's inevitable that we will come away feeling rather stingy. We all have limited resources. Just how much can we afford to give to a life-sucking baby?

I'm certainly not going to argue with the notion that motherhood costs us something. Of course it does—physically, financially, emotionally, and spiritually. Sarah Reinhard knows this too, and these pages, she offers us encouragement and a means of "feeding" ourselves throughout pregnancy. Gently, she nudges us away from worldly ways of counting costs and toward a more generous and grateful attitude about the privilege of nurturing new life, growing within.

Sarah's realistic and yet positive approach reminds me of Blessed John Paul II's take on siblings and motherhood. Our beloved pope challenged American parents toward greater generosity.

"Americans are known for generosity to your children. And what is the best gift you can give your children? I say to you: Give them brothers and sisters."

Pregnancy is a gift? Children are a gift? These are poetic words, but they don't fail to acknowledge the trials involved in answering the call to raise a family. Like any gift we offer, like anything we do out of love, pregnancy, childbirth, and raising a family require personal sacrifice.

What pregnancy and motherhood cost us can be calculated—in lost hours of sleep, grocery bills, and tuition payments; but can we place a price tag on the gift of a unique and immortal human soul, created in the image and likeness of God?

Can we quantify the "growing up" that happens when a woman becomes a mother? Can we add up the benefits to our families, our communities, and ourselves, when we bring the gift of new life to the world? Can we calculate the kind of real growth, the kind of work toward holiness, and the kind of blessing that takes when a woman follows Mary's example and says Yes to motherhood?

I don't think we can. We can only live it. And, thanks be to God for the privilege to do so, for nine months, and a lifetime to come.

Danielle Bean

Acknowledgments

ACKNOWLEDGING ALL THE HELP I RECEIVED WILL BE impossible, but I'm going to take a stab at it, all the same. After all, that's part of my job!

First, to the contributors who graciously and generously shared their hearts: thank-you.

To the beta readers who not only made kind comments about the ugly first draft, but also encouraged me not to burn it, including Ali Arend, Jen Fitz, Shelly Kelly, Brittany Shoots-Reinhard, and Walt Staples: thank-you.

To Jen Fitz, for keeping me accountable and sending me quite a few huzzahs and even offering things up so that I could get this thing off my desk: thank-you.

To Lisa Hendey, for your prayers, support, encouragement, and laughs as I journeyed through the writing of this book: thank-you.

To my dear sister-of-the-heart, Ali, for taking the kids, not laughing at me when I complained *again*, and for listening to my rants *again*: thank-you.

To Mom Ann, for pulling mommy rank as needed and baking with abandon: thank-you.

To Susie, for being an inspiration and a light for me in the dark days of wondering why I bother to write: thank-you.

To Kristi McDonald, for making the task of working with an editor more like drinking tea over the phone with a younger sister than a harrowing artistic process: thank-you.

To Bob Hamma, for being so kind, supportive, and humorous (in your low-key, humble way): thank-you.

To the other people at Ave Maria Press, whose names I either don't know or didn't think to name, who have dealt with far better than me, but make me feel like a princess anyway: thank-you.

To my Bob, for all the usual reasons, but also because you still smile when I call myself a writer, for being so good at listening to the Holy Spirit, and for so often being the voice of God to me: thank-you and I love you.

And finally, to the many saints and angels I called upon in my desperate attempts to make sense out of the words scrambling around in my brain, and most especially to Mama Mary: thank-you.

Notes

1. "Saint Gerard Majella," Saints.SQPN.com, accessed January 31, 2012, http://saints.sqpn.com/saint-gerard-majella/.

2. Glade B. Curtis and Judith Schuler, *Your Pregnancy Week by Week*, 6th ed. (Cambridge, MA: Da Capo Press, 2007), 101.

3. Ibid., 117.

4. Ibid., 130.

5. Ibid., 132.

6. Louis de Montfort, "Prayer of Renewal of Baptismal Promises," accessed online at http://acta-sanctorum.blogspot.com/2010/01/prayer-of-renewal-of-baptismal-promises.html on 3/16/12.

7. Curtis and Schuler, 143.

8. Ibid., 156.

9. William Sears, Martha Sears, and Linda Hughey Holt, *The Pregnancy Book: Month-by-Month, Everything You Need to Know from America's Baby Experts* (New York: Little, Brown, 1997), 118.

10. Ibid.

11. Curtis and Schuler, 173.

12. John Paul II, *Familiaris Consortio* (On the Role of the Christian Family in the Modern World), 22 November 1981, www.vatican.va/holy_father/john_paul_ii/apost_exhortations/documentshf_jp-ii_exh_19811122_familiaris-consortio_en.html.

13. Curtis and Schuler, 184.

14. Ibid., 186.

15. "Mary's Gardens," accessed February 22, 2012, http://campus.udayton.edu/mary /resources/m_garden/marygardensmain.html.

16. Ann Ball, "Litany to the Heart of Jesus," in *Encyclopedia of Catholic Devotions and Practices* (Huntington, IN: Our Sunday Visitor, 2002), 315–316.

17. Jerome, "Commentary on Isaiah," The Crossroads Initiative, accessed January 31, 2012, http://crossroadsinitiative.com/library_article /257/Ignorance_of_Scripture_is_Ignorance_of_Christ_St._Jerome.html.

18. Rosary Army, www.rosaryarmy.com.

19. Saint's Name Generator, accessed February 22, 2012, http://jenniferfulwiler.com /saints. (This is one of several sites.)

20. Surgeworks, Inc., "Morning Offering" Prayer 2000+ Catholic Prayers by Divine Office.org, accessed January 31, 2011, http://itunes.apple.com/us/app/prayer-2000+-catholic-prayers/id307757516?mt=8.

21. Robert M. Hamma, *Together at Baptism: Preparing for the Celebration of Your Child's Baptism* (Notre Dame, IN: Ave Maria Press, 1994), 20.

22. Ron Lewinski, *Guide for Sponsors* (Chicago: Liturgy Training Publications, 1993), 10–11.

23. Hamma, 52.

About the Contributors

Karen Murphy Corr (p. 145) is a freelance writer and former journalist living in beautiful British Columbia, Canada, with her husband of nineteen years, Philip Corr. They are raising baby George's three big brothers and big sister and just welcomed his little sister in 2011.

Jennifer Fitz (p. 103) is a homeschool mom of four, catechist, writer, and accountant. She writes for the Catholic Writers' Guild blog at http://blog.catholicwritersguild.com and on her personal blog, www.jenniferfitz.wordpress. Her latest project is a book of support, encouragement, and practical advice for parents struggling with the decision to homeschool. She writes, "I absolutely love homeschooling. But that doesn't mean it's the best choice for every family. Let go of the guilt, and be the parent God made you to be."

Jane Lebak (p. 89) is the author of *Seven Archangels: Annihilation* (Double-Edged Publishing, 2008), *The Boys Upstairs* (MuseItUp, 2010), and over fifty shorter pieces. She blogs at http://philangelus.wordpress.com and maintains a website for parents carrying to term after a diagnosis fatal to the baby at www.janelebak.com/cct/index.html. Her first novel, *The Guardian*, will be reissued by Written World Communications in 2012.

Mary DeTurris Poust (p. 27) is an author, columnist, blogger, and public speaker who has focused on Catholic issues for more than twenty-five years. She is the author of four books: *Walking Together: Discovering the Catholic Tradition of Spiritual Friendship, The Essential Guide to Catholic Prayer and the Mass, The Complete Idiot's Guide to the Catholic Catechism*, and *Parenting a Grieving Child: Helping Children Find Faith, Hope and Healing after the Loss of a Loved One*. Mary blogs regularly at *OSV Daily Take* and at her own blog, *Not Strictly Spiritual*. Her monthly column "Life Lines" has been published in *Catholic New York* since 2001. She lives in upstate New York with her husband Dennis and their three children. For more information, visit her website at www.marydeturrispoust.com.

Dorian Speed (p. 163) is a writer and former teacher who lives with her husband and three children near Houston. Her work has appeared in a variety of print and online publications, and she blogs about faith, culture, education, and family at scrutinies.net. She is currently the web editor for the literary magazine, *Dappled Things*.

Leticia Velasquez (p. 65) is the author of *A Special Mother is Born*, an inspirational collection of stories from Catholic parents of special-needs children, and is a contributor to *Encyclopedia of Catholic Social Thought* and the award-winning *Stories for the Homeschool Heart*. She writes three blogs: *Catholic Media Review, Cause of Our Joy*, and the Pro-Life Blog award-winning *Causa Nostrae Laetitiae*. In 2008 she co-founded KIDS (Keep Infants with Down Syndrome) to raise awareness of the 92 percent abortion rate of babies with Down syndrome. She has appeared on EWTN, Canadian television, and on various radio programs including NPR, *The Drew Mariani Show*, and the *Son Rise Morning Show*. She is a correspondent for the *National Catholic Register*, a contributor to *MercatorNet*, *Catholic Lane*, and *Catholic Online*, and she is a columnist for CatholicMom.com. She, her husband of twenty years, and their four daughters live in rural Connecticut.

Kate Wicker (p. 13) is a wife and mom of littles, journalist, speaker, and expert in hazardous-waste removal. A senior writer and health columnist for *Faith & Family* magazine, Kate is also the author of *Weightless: Making Peace with Your Body*. Kate has written for numerous regional and national media, including *Atlanta Parent, Catholic Exchange, CatholicMom.com, Catholic News Agency, Children's Ministry Magazine, Crisis Magazine, Family Fun, Fathers For Good, Pregnancy, Pittsburgh Parent*, and *Woman's Day*. In addition, Kate is a regular voice on the Faith & Family Live! podcast. She's also been a guest on a myriad of other Catholic programming such as the Among Women podcast, *Kresta in the Afternoon* radio show, the *Busted Halo Show*, the *Catholics Next Door*, and EWTN's *Son Rise Morning Show*. Visit her website at katewicker.com.

SARAH A. REINHARD is a popular Catholic writer, blogger, and contributor to such sites as *CatholicMom.com, Integrated Catholic Life, New Evangelizers*, and *Amazing Catechists*. She produces a weekly segment on Mary for the *iPadre, Catholic Foodie,* and *Uncommon Sense* podcasts.

In addition to serving as editor of her parish's publications, ministry scheduler, and odds-and-ends parish support, Reinhard is the author of five books for Catholic families and writes a monthly column in the Diocese of Columbus's *The Catholic Times*. She also contributes a weekly column on the Catholic Writers Guild's blog. Reinhard holds a master's degree in marketing and communications and has worked for many years in corporate and nonprofit organizations. She lives in central Ohio with her husband and three children. Visit Reinhard online at *SnoringScholar.com*.